T0211752

Medical Dominance

Studies in Society

Medical Dominance

The division of labour in Australian health care

EVAN WILLIS

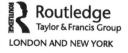

Routledge
Taylor & Francis Group

LONDON AND NEW YORK

First published 1989 by Allen & Unwin

Published 2020 by Routledge
2 Park Square, Milton Park, Abingdon, Oxon OX14 4RN
605 Third Avenue, New York, NY 10017

Routledge is an imprint of the Taylor & Francis Group, an informa business

National Library of Australia
Cataloguing-in-Publication entry:
Willis, Evan, 1952–
   Medical dominance: the division of labour in Australian health care.

   2nd ed.
   Bibliography.
   Includes index.

   1. Medical care—Australia. 2. Physicians—Australia.
   3. Medical personnel—Australia. I. Title. (Series: Studies in society
   (Sydney, N.S.W.)).

362.1'0994

Library of Congress Catalog Card Number: 83–70839

Set in 10/11 Times by Graphicraft Typesetters Limited, Hong Kong

ISBN—13: 9780043600702 (pbk)

Contents

Abbreviations   vii

Preface   ix

1 Introduction   1

2 Theoretical considerations   8

3 The rise of medicine: the pre-scientific era   36

4 Technical and political process in the rise of
scientific medicine   61

5 The subordination of midwifery   92

6 The limitation of optometry   125

7 The exclusion of chiropractic   162

8 Conclusion   201

Postscript: the politics of medical dominance   217

Methodological appendix   221

Bibliography   226

Index   245

For Miranda

Abbreviations

ABS	Australian Bureau of Statistics
ACA	Australian Chiropractors' Association
ACO	Australian College of Optometry
AJO	Australian/Australasian Journal of Optometry
AMA	Australian Medical Association
AMJ	Australian Medical Journal
AMJWOG	Australian Manufacturing Jewellers, Watchmakers and Opticians Gazette
AOA	Australian Optometrical Association
APA	Australian Physiotherapy Association
ATNA	Australian Trained Nurses Association
BMA	British Medical Association
CPD	Commonwealth Parliamentary Debates
CPP	Commonwealth Parliamentary Papers
CSO	Chief Secretary's Office Files—held at Public Records Office
ICC	International College of Chiropractic
IMJA	Intercolonial Medical Journal of Australia
LTLMS	La Trobe Library Manuscript
MBV	Medical Board of Victoria
MDA	Medical Defence Association
MJA	Medical Journal of Australia
MMA	Melbourne Medical Association
MOA	Master Opticians' Association
MSV	Medical Society of Victoria
NSWPP	New South Wales Parliamentary Papers
OERS	Optometrical Education Reform Society
OPSM	Optical Prescriptions Spectacle Makers Pty Ltd
ORB	Optometrical Registration Board
OS	Ophthalmological Society
PIT	Preston Institute of Technology
RACO	Royal Australian College of Ophthalmologists
RMIT	Royal Melbourne Institute of Technology
RVTNA	Royal Victorian Trained Nurses Association
SMT	Spinal Manipulative Therapy

UCA	United Chiropractors' Association
VCO	Victorian College of Optometry
VGG	Victorian Government Gazette
VIC	Victorian Institute of Colleges
VOA	Victorian Optometrical Association
VPD	Victorian Parliamentary Debates
VPP	Victorian Parliamentary Papers
VTNA	Victorian Trained Nurses Association

Preface

No intellectual effort occurs in isolation and it is appropriate to express due thanks to the many people who have assisted with this study, while of course retaining full responsibility for the end result. Foremost among these people are my wife Johanna Wyn and Pat O'Malley who supervised the original PhD thesis research on which this book is based. Both contributed enormously in personal supportive terms and in critically reviewing and discussing the research as it progressed.

I am grateful to a number of individuals who assisted with the research in their organisational capacities: Miss Cecily Close of the Melbourne University Archives; Mr Daryl Guest and Mr Charles Wright of the Australian Optometrical Association; Dr Andries Kleynhans and Mrs Maureen Ellis of the International College of Chiropractic; Mr Rod Smith of the Public Records Office; Miss Ann Tovell of the AMA Archives; and the staff of the La Trobe (State) Library. John Nathan kindly made available his father's personal papers for study.

Other people commented critically and suggested improvements on the manuscripts for which I am grateful. These include Rod Andrew, Bill Foddy, Neville Hicks, John McKinlay and Ron Wild. Sue Stevenson expertly typed the manuscript. Also to be acknowledged is the assistance provided by my students in 'Sociology of Health and Illness' courses from 1978 to 1982 at Monash University with whom many of the ideas incorporated in the book were argued and thrashed out in a stimulating yet critical environment.

Preface to the second edition

The opportunity for an afterword is appreciated in view of the way that the concept of medical dominance has become part of the discourse of health care policy analysis in Australia.

The second edition is different from the first in two important respects. The conclusion has been substantially rewritten to bring developments in the social structure of health care delivery up to date. It also assesses the continuing relevance of medical dominance theory against other explanations which have been proposed to understand changes in health care delivery. The other change from the first edition is the addition of a postscript on the politics of medical dominance. The study hopefully stands as a piece of scholarship; this postscript addresses the more political question of what medical dominance means for people's health.

I would like to express thanks to a number of people who have provided the sort of intellectual environment in which this work has been developed. Foremost amongst these have been Jeanne Daly and Lynne Ham. I am also grateful for support to Ken Dempsey, Neville Hicks, Ian MacDonald, John McKinlay, Bryan Turner, Rosemary Wearing and Maria Zadoroznyj.

1 Introduction

This book analyses the production of health services through the complex arrangement of healing tasks that is socially organised into a structure known as the division of labour. The process of health care delivery has become extremely specialised so that in the course of receiving health care a person is likely to come into contact with a variety of health personnel. Such personnel are differentiated primarily by the occupations they represent but also by other factors such as gender, ethnicity and class. The division of labour in which these health personnel provide health care is a complex one constituting the social structure of health care delivery. The attempted explanation for this social structure provides the central analytical focus of this book.

Two features of the division of labour in health care are immediately apparent. One is its hierarchical nature, the other its domination by one occupation: the medical profession. That the division of labour in health care has become highly complex and specialised is beyond doubt. From censuses for instance it can be shown that in 1871 doctors constituted 33 per cent of the Victorian health workforce whereas by 1976 this figure had dropped to only 12 per cent. The Census of 1911 recognised only thirteen categories of health personnel, whereas the Federal Health Department in its *Handbook on Health Manpower* recognised no less than 105 different health occupations in 1980.

The hierarchical nature of the social structure of health care can be represented in Table 1.1 (overleaf). The division of labour can be differentiated on two different though interrelated bases. One is by occupation forming the occupational division of labour, the other by gender forming the sexual division of labour. The two together result in an hierarchical structure entailing huge disparities in average income.

The other feature of the division of labour in health care is the phenomenon of medical dominance. The term 'medicine' it is relevant to note, is commonly used in at least three different ways: firstly to a body of knowledge (in this study this will be referred to as scientific medicine); secondly as an institution, the medical system (in this study

Table 1.1   Division of labour in health care

	% Total	% Women	$ p.a.
Doctors, Dentists	8.1	12.4	67 000
Admin. and Exec.	1.2	36.5	22 000
Pharm., Therapists	3.3	60.0	16 000
Technician, Social workers	3.6	60.0	16 000
Nurses	34.9	95.0	14 000
Clerical	12.7	91.6	10 500
Trades, Process workers	6.4	20.4	10 500
Nurse aide attendants	11.8	75.7	9 200
Kitchen, Laundry, Cleaning	14.8	81.1	9 200
Unclassified	3.2	—	—

Note: Total—4.6 per cent of total workforce (there are also workers in other industries whose output is used by health services). Seventy-five per cent of total are women.
Sources: Workforce—1971 Census unpublished tabulations Income—Unions etc. Figures relate to early 1981.

the term health system is preferred). Thirdly it has been used to refer to an occupation, the medical profession. In this study the term medicine will be used only in this last sense. Medicine dominates the health division of labour economically, politically, socially and intellectually. This phenomenon of medical dominance is the key feature of the production of health care in Australian society and the central analytical focus in explaining the social structure and organisation of health care.

Medical dominance in the health division of labour is sustained at three different levels: over its own work; over the work of others; and in the wider health sphere. At the level of control over the medical profession's own work medical dominance is denoted as *autonomy*. Medicine is not subject to direction and evaluation by other health occupations. Medicine, as Freidson (1970a: 127) argues occupies 'a legally or otherwise formally created position, one which entails a monopoly over a set of services and accessories required'. This is the result he argues, of the exclusive right granted to doctors to penetrate the body, physically by surgery or chemically by drugs.

Not only has medicine gained the right to deny the legitimacy of evaluation by others, but it has also gained control over the work of other health occupations. This second level of analysis denotes a relationship of *authority* over other health occupations. For many health occupations this authority is direct and involves the supervising and directing the work of others. However, even those occupations which are outside the direct evaluation and thence control of medicine, are nonetheless likely to be indirectly controlled by the involvement of doctors in the formal organisation of their work. This can occur either by medical representation on their registration boards or by the denial of legitimacy through medical opposition.

Historically medicine has been able to define the conditions under which it will recognise and legitimate other health occupations. These recognised occupations are defined as being of two sorts, 'ancillary' personnel and 'other clinical vocations'. Recognition of these other health workers and 'professional association' (ie working with) was defined by the Medical Services Review Committee of the Australian Medical Association (AMA), the main occupational association of doctors, as being dependent upon a formal agreement based on ten points. These cover aspects such as level of training, vocational titles, homogeneity of other occupations, and their knowledge basis. On the relationship with medicine, any direct association must be under the control and direction of doctors, the code of ethics must be compatible with that of medicine and the occupation must agree not to mislead the public on what it is qualified to treat, or on its relationship with medicine (MJA, 17 June 1967: 93). Occupations which cannot meet these ten conditions have been opposed by medicine and legitimacy traditionally denied them.

The issue of legitimacy raises the third level of analysis at which medical dominance is sustained in the wider society. This will be denoted by the term *medical sovereignty*. At this level medicine is dominant in relations between the health sector and the wider society; doctors are institutionalised experts on all matters relating to health. The effect of this is that state patronage for other health occupations has been historically contingent upon medical approval or at least acquiescence. Registration has traditionally been on terms acceptable to medicine or not at all.

The division of labour in health care has not been the subject of a great deal of research. As Atkinson et al. (1977: 244), argue the study of professional occupations 'is rich in theoretical discussion and survey material but poorly served with more detailed data', particularly involving the case history approach of the relationship between health occupations. The need, as Larkin (1978: 856) argues is that the study of the division of labour 'should be rooted in a more historical sociology of medical occupations'. Specifically the relationship between the class structure and the medical division of labour needs to be historically analysed as both Freidson (1970a: 3) and McKinlay (1977) indicate.

Even then, much of what research has been done has substantial limitations and tends not to adequately analyse the complex historical process which occurred. Most accounts either operate from a consensus perspective (eg Etzioni, 1969; Greenfield, 1969; Moore, 1970) and thus tend to underplay the very real and bitter conflicts which frequently occurred, or alternatively have focused conceptually on the notion of roles (eg Davies, 1979b). The latter approach tends to be ahistorical as Connell (1979a: 16) has argued, presented more statically than the dynamic historical development of the work of different occupations.

This book by contrast analyses the division of labour in health care as a process based upon conflict; a struggle between occupations and between the sexes, not so much over occupational roles but over occupational territory or task domains. An occupational territory, viewed this way is an area of health knowledge and healing tasks based upon that knowledge over which an occupation claims competence. For example, an issue of current controversy within the health system is the suggested proposal to limit the taking of X-rays to radiologists and radiographers and not to allow chiropractors who have taken X-rays for many years to continue to do so. This debate is about the question of 'on whose occupational territory does the taking of X-rays fall'. The definition of occupational territories is an ongoing historical process. As Bucher and Strauss (1961) argue, formal occupational territories are established by legislation, and the boundaries of these are produced and reproduced in political struggle with occupations attempting to defend or extend their relative position.

Therefore the division of labour in health care must be studied historically in terms of a continuing struggle over appropriate occupational territories. As Larkin (1978: 853) has argued, the phenomenon of medical dominance 'is a shorthand concept for a complex historical process of the establishment of control'. To analyse this historical process, which is in large part the result of the dialectical relationship between two factors, a materialist approach is adopted. One of these is the material conditions of Australian society; that is, capitalism as the system of productive relationships involving generalised commodity production and private property which has given rise to a polarised class structure. The second component of this relationship is the ideology of the dominant class in Australian society.

Using this analysis, the traditional explanation for the division of labour in health care is challenged. This 'technological determinist' argument explains the position of occupations in the division of labour by the differing relationships to and control over that knowledge and the technology based upon it (eg Mechanic, 1976; Sax, 1972). Medicine dominates the health division of labour according to this explanation because it controls the knowledge upon which healing is based. The division of labour can be seen as the expression of knowledge relationships in an hierarchical form. In this book by contrast it is argued that the role of medical knowledge and technology has been overstated. Rather it is argued, the development of a specialised division of labour in health care is related to the preservation of control over health care by the medical profession, the occupation which dominates the health division of labour. Differentiation in the division of labour has occurred in such a way as to allow medicine to retain its dominant position.

Important to this explanation is its concern with the wider politico-economic context in which differentiation in the division of labour occurs. McKinlay (1977: 464) outlines four separate levels of analysis of what he calls the 'business of medicine', arranged in order of their determining influence. At the highest level is financial and industrial capital and their effect on the conduct of medicine. The second level is the capitalist state with its emphases on legitimation and the provision of opportunities for capital accumulation. At the third level is medicine itself; how medical activity is conducted within the constraints of the two higher levels. Finally the level of the public as patients constitutes the fourth level. As McKinlay shows, most medical sociology concerns itself at the level of medicine and the interaction between medicine and the public. What this study attempts to do by contrast is to examine the other influences, particularly the state upon the division of labour in the health system.

Specifically it is argued that the development of medical dominance cannot be adequately understood without an examination of the changing nature of Australian capitalism. The major change to be considered here, which provides an essential backcloth to the development of the division of labour in health care, was the transition from laissez-faire to monopoly capitalism. Although this change is not greatly analysed in the literature and took a different form in Australia from other countries, its major effects were a substantial growth in the role of the state, particularly in the welfare (including health) arena, a general trend towards the commodification of areas of human activity and the development of new forms of ideology to legitimate the economic changes which took place. Only by examining the effects of these politico-economic changes within the health sector can the development of the division of labour be adequately understood.

Where the state is particularly important is in the provision of licensing laws. These provide a legal foundation for the division of labour. Licensing is a form of legal protection for the occupational territories of various health occupations from competitors. The state, in other words, provides those occupations with statutory registration in the form of licensing laws, a means of self defense against encroachment upon their means of livelihood. As Bucher and Strauss (1961) argue, licensing laws are the historical deposits of the exercise of power and authority. The struggle for licensing and over the content of the legislation by various occupations is a major process to be analysed. This process of struggle over occupational territory and registration however can only be understood by reference to the other levels of analysis, in particular financial and industrial capital. The division of labour has evolved through struggle, both class struggle (inter and intra class conflict) and also through a struggle between the sexes. Class and state patronage of medicine have enabled its dominance in the health field to be achieved and sustained.

The argument of the book is laid out as follows. Chapter two provides the theoretical foundations upon which the subsequent historical analysis is based and those readers with little interest in these issues are invited to pass on to the subsequent chapters. In analysing the division of labour and the phenomenon of medical dominance there are two aspects to consider: one is its *production* (how it was created originally); the other its *reproduction* (how it has been defended and extended over time). The two are facets of the same historical process and separable for analytic purposes only as they overlap temporally to a considerable extent. The production of medical dominance is examined in chapters three and four, tracing the rise of the medical profession to a position of dominance within the Victorian health system. Its reproduction is considered by analysing the different modes of domination which different health occupations historically have experienced in their relationship to medicine. For each mode of domination one health occupation has been chosen and the development of its relationship to medicine traced.

Subordination is the first mode of domination to be considered in chapter five with midwifery as the chosen occupation. These occupations work under the direct control of doctors, are overwhelmingly female and relate the sexual division of labour to the occupational division of labour. The second mode to be considered, in chapter six is *limitation*. These occupations such as dentistry and optometry have not had direct medical control but more indirect control through legal restriction on their occupational territories and medical presence on their registration boards. Optometry has been chosen to illustrate this mode of domination. Finally *exclusion* is analysed in chapter seven. Excluded occupations have traditionally been denied official legitimacy in the form of licensing and have come to be known as 'alternative' medicine as a result. Chiropractic is the chosen example here.

It should be noted that other modes of domination are possible though not historically important in Australian context. For example, 'incorporation' occurs where occupations are absorbed into medicine and lose their separate identity, for example osteopathy in many parts of United States (though not in Australia). Finally in chapter eight the argument is drawn together and some of the implications of findings discussed.

This book is basically a revised and shortened version of my PhD thesis entitled 'The Division of Labour in Health Care' (Monash University, 1982). Further theoretical and empirical details may be found there.

2 Theoretical considerations

In this chapter the theoretical framework for the study as a whole is set out. The aim is to construct the scaffolding on which the study is based. The intention it should be noted is not to specify a priori what is to be found in evidence but to provide a basis for ordering the mass of historical data utilised.

The main thrust of this chapter is to theorise the notion 'medical dominance' in the health division of labour. As indicated previously medical dominance is sustained at three different levels: over medicine's own work, over the work of other health occupations and in the wider societal sphere. Dominance at each level can be represented by the concepts of autonomy, authority and medical sovereignty. This chapter seeks to locate theoretically each of those notions. In order to theorise the phenomenon of medical dominance adequately it is necessary to consider the inter-relationship between four factors in particular: occupation, class, gender, and the capitalist state. Finally in this chapter the division of labour itself is analysed.

Autonomy and professionalism

Control over medicine's own work, the first level at which medical dominance is sustained, is based upon the claim to professionalism, here viewed as an occupational ideology legitimating autonomy. Ideology as used here is a complex and contradictory set of ideas, representations, actions and practives grounded in social relations. Importantly it has a material force being grounded in actual concrete practices reflecting the major social relations in a society. The argument made is that professionalism can only be understood in terms of class and gender relations at the level of the state.

The conceptual confusion with the terms 'profession', 'professionalisation' and 'professionalism' has been considerable. Clearly the phenomenon must be studied historically. The professions as we know them today, originated with the advent of capitalism especially in the nineteenth century (Laslett, 1971: 52), and their expansion provided a link between the educational system and the occupational order (Schudson, 1980: 177).

Their emergence soon attracted the attention of social scientists who tended to focus on two questions: to what extent were professions a unique development in the division of labour; and secondly what role did this new occupational group perform in modern industrial, capitalist society? Their answers varied. For Marx (1969), professions were of secondary derivative character because they were unproductive. For Durkheim (1957) by contrast, professions were a means of regulation and integration in modern societies characterised by organic solidarity and a redress against excessive individualism. Weber (1968) incorporated their development into his view of class as market capacity.

The tradition of study of professions which developed in the twentieth century reflected a Durkheimian legacy. As Johnson (1972) has shown, two related approaches can be distinguished. One became concerned with definitional issues (eg Greenwood, 1957) about what 'traits' define a profession and how far along the process of professionalisation various occupations are. These studies in Johnson's mind 'litter the field' (1972: 10) and have proved largely sterile. The other approach has been a functionalist one, dominated by Parsons (1964, 1968), which stressed the functionality of professions for the maintenance of the social order. For both trait and functionalist theories, professionalisation was a positive aspect of modernisation and a relief from what was seen as Weber's gloomy analysis of increasing rationalisation and bureaucratisation in modern societies. In this tradition is the classic work of Carr-Saunders and Wilson (1933), who argued that professions functioned as a bulwark against threats to the social order, in particular against the growth of large scale bureaucratic organisations.

A much needed fillip to the study of the professions was provided in the 1970s by Freidson (1970a, 1970b) and Johnson (1972). Both were explicitly critical of the traditional approach, insisting that professions and professionalism were concerned with power and control. A powerful critique was directed at the traditional approach. The attributes used were shown to be marks of an occupational group which had successfully attained a privileged position. The process of professionalisation which the traditional approach stressed was shown to be ahistorical. The traditional approach furthermore accepted the profession's own reality rather than investigating it. Furthermore the traditional approach did not attempt to locate the power of the professions in the wider societal context at the level of the state. Such an explanation requires a class analysis of the professions in capitalist society. The Durkheimian legacy had led the sociology of the professions away from a concern with class structure and formation, as

Parry and Parry (1976) have shown. Unlike both Marx and Weber, classes receive little attention in Durkheim's work, and this is reproduced not only in the traditional approach but also to a considerable extent in that of Freidson and Johnson also.

For Freidson, the major distinction between a profession and other occupations is the legitimate and organised autonomy possessed by that profession. Such autonomy gives the profession an occupational monopoly which ensures a position of dominance in a division of labour (Freidson, 1977: 24). Such autonomy and control is based in theoretical terms on dual foundations. One is esoteric knowledge, the other recognition and protection of that knowledge by state patronage. Medicine he argues, has a unique position originating from two sources. One of these is the state itself. He argues that 'the foundation on which the analysis of a profession must be based is its relationship to the ultimate source of power and authority in modern society—the state. In the case of medicine, much, though by no means all, of the profession's strength is based on legally supported monopoly over practice' (Freidson, 1970a: 83). The second factor is the support of unidentified strategic elites:

> A profession attains and maintains its position by virtue of the protection and patronage of some strategic elite segment of society which has been persuaded that there is some special value in its work. Its position is thus secured by the political and economic influence of the elite which sponsors it—an influence that drives competing occupations out of the same area of work, that discourages others by virtue of the competitive advantages conferred on the chosen occupation and that requires still others to be subordinated to the profession. (Freidson, 1970b: 72–73)

Yet this insightful analysis does not enable the source of autonomy to be located. As McKinlay (1977: 465–466) has shown, Freidson leaves unaddressed many of the questions raised such as: Who are these strategic elites? What is their relationship to the state? What is the nature of this relationship between the professions and the state? What class interests are behind the term 'professionalisation'? What special value does the work of doctors have for this group?

The answer to these questions lies in the analysis of class structures. Following Frankenberg (1974), I will argue that it is most useful to see the elites which Freidson mentions as a class. In this case, this is the dominant class, defined by private ownership and control of productive resources.

In his early work, Johnson (1972) also focuses on power and control. He argues that professionalism must be seen as one form of occupational control, and a subtype of 'collegiate control' (mateship?). It is akin to the Parsonian notion of control by a 'company of equals'. Professionalism for Johnson is the end point of a process of professionalisation which only a few occupations have historically achieved. However as Johnson himself later recognises (1977), he fails to identify the conditions which give rise to the various forms of occupational control he outlines and to locate this classification within an adequate theory of class relations. The furthest he goes is to argue that the success of an occupational group depends upon their access to 'wider bases of social power'.

The advances made by Freidson and Johnson however, stimulated new interest in the sociology of the professions and their stress on the need for a conflict perspective to examine relations of power and authority in specific historical contexts led to the emergence of several sociological histories of the medical profession itself (Berlant, 1975; Parry and Parry, 1976; Larson, 1977). While all provide excellent insights into the nature of the control medicine has over its own work, particularly Larson, they all have inadequate conceptions of class relations in their analyses. This does not allow them to adequately resolve the issues of the theoretical status of professionalism and its relationship with class and political orders. The first two of these employ an explicitly Weberian perspective adopting and applying Weber's analysis of class formation to medicine itself. Berlant (1975) focuses more on the monopolisation strategy itself while Parry and Parry (1976) stress collective social mobility as the result of closure and monopolisation. Both consider that professionalism is an occupational strategy which can be understood only in relation to the development and maintenance of the class structure. Yet problems exist with the class analyses made in both these accounts. Berlant (1975: 305) for instance stresses the importance of the rise of state power to the success of medicine in the United States yet does no more than indicate the need for class analyses to explain this. Medicine was successful he argues because of a 'compatible constellation of interests' between medicine and 'powerful social groups' or elites without proceeding to examine the basis for this constellation of interests.

For Parry and Parry (1976) professionalism is a middle class strategy aimed at upward social mobility of the occupation collectively. Such a process is important to class formation, or what they call (drawing on Giddens, 1973) class structuration. While stressing, the centrality of class theory to an analysis of professionalism, the utility of their analysis is limited, as with Berlant, by the class theory adopted. Based upon a stratificationist approach, it is basically a variety of embourgeoisement theory, and confuses changing indices of status with alterations in the class structure itself.

For Larson (1977) the 'professional project', besides these efforts to control markets and gain status through the 'collective mobility project', has a third component, an ideological one. According to Larson, what professions have in common is an occupational ideology —a claim to autonomy (1977: 219). The collective mobility project aimed at enhancing status for instance, has important ideological consequences in blinding the facts of relative subordination and powerlessness by the professionals themselves, thus pacifying them. Yet a rise in status does not alter the location in a system of class relations she argues. While her analysis of the ideology of professionalism is a useful one, she fails to specify the conditions under which that claim to autonomy is sustained. Like Berlant she points to the possibilities of doing this (in her case with a Gramscian analysis) but does not proceed herself.

Mention should also be made here of two other works relevant to the present discussion. The first of these is the major recent account of similar processes being examined in this study by Pensabene, entitled *The Rise of the Medical Practitioner in Victoria* (1980). An economic historian by training, Pensabene's analysis does not examine sociological issues in detail but is based upon detailed original historical analysis which is drawn upon for purposes of secondary analysis in this book. The book traces the rise of medicine from a low status and divided occupation in the 1860s to a high status and politically unified occupation by the 1930s. Based implicitly on Friedson's work it suffers from similar inadequacies, in particular the failure to locate the process within a theory of class relations. Much is made of changing power and status, yet these concepts remain untheorised and unrelated to the changing nature of the Australian capitalist state. Two other criticisms are worth mentioning here since the interpretations put upon some of the data provided by Pensabene are different in this study from the original. One is that despite his emphasis on disunity within the profession, Pensabene downplays the segmentation of medicine particularly in the twentieth century. Secondly Pensabene locates the basis of medical power in technological determinist terms. Changes in medical science, it is argued, raised the community's perception of the skills of medical practitioners (Pensabene, 1980: 177). In the political sphere the use of power elite and interest group theory diverts attention away from the role of the capitalist state (see Navarro, 1976: 186–92).

The other relevant work is that of Navarro (1976) which stresses class relations and the state to the neglect of the specific character of professionalism. Writing from an orthodox Marxist perspective, Navarro is little interested in the phenomenon of professionalism; indeed it has no relevance to his analysis, being of a secondary and derivative character. For Navarro, professions are a reflection of the class structure found in the wider society and have no independent analytic existence. While acknowledging the importance of Navarro's work in general, I would argue that this also represents an insufficient explanation for the phenomenon of medical dominance. Despite his rejection of economic determinism and claim to dialecticism, Navarro's analysis tends to be reductionist. In particular the role of ideology is undeveloped in this work.

Health occupations and the class structure

In order to provide a theory about medical dominance it is necessary to locate the medical profession within the class structure of advanced capitalist societies. Since most analyses of the division of labour stress its occupational basis, usually in terms of roles (eg Davies, 1979b), and I have argued here for the centrality of its class basis, the relationship between occupation and class must be considered. Distributive, stratificationist approaches to social class take occupation (or more particularly occupational status) along with income as the empirical referents of class (eg Broom et al., 1979). These social characteristics are used to locate class boundaries (see Parkin, 1974).

In this study by contrast, following Wright (1980b) the relationship between class and occupation is viewed differently. Whereas stratificationist approaches have tended to view 'occupation' and 'class' as occupying essentially the same theoretical terrain, here they are seen as occupying different theoretical terrains.

> Occupations are understood as positions defined within the *technical* relations of production; classes on the other hand are defined by the *social* relations of production. Occupations are thus defined by an array of technical functions or activities: . . . a doctor transforms sick people into healthy people . . . Classes on the other hand can only be defined in terms of their social relationship to other classes, or in more precise terms by their location within the social relations of production. (Wright, 1980b: 177; emphasis in original)

Therefore classes cannot be defined as clusters of occupations as they occupy basically different theoretical spaces. Occupations form a part of the technical division of labour; classes form a part of the social division of labour. The argument to be made here is that the two exist in a dialectical relationship in which the social (class) has primacy over the technical (occupation).

In order to locate the professions in general and the medical profession in particular within the class structure of advanced capitalist societies, a variety of neo-Marxist theory known as Marxist structuralism is drawn upon. This locates professions as part of the new middle class. Many writers have commented upon the lack of a systematic treatment of class in Marx's work. Attempts to draw out a theory of class structure from Marx's works have led to great disagreements among writers, both Marxist and non-Marxist. The most frequent criticism has been that Marx failed to predict the rise and continued importance of an intermediary class grouping, which, far from being a temporary phenomenon of capitalism only to wither under the impact of polarisation and proletarianisation, has remained important with the evolution of capitalism (eg Dahrendorf, 1959; Giddens, 1973).

Recently, however, there have appeared several attempts to theorise about the location of this intermediary class grouping in Marxist terms (Poulantzas, 1973, 1975; Carchedi, 1977; Wright, 1980a, 1980b). Although there are considerable differences between them as to exactly how this intermediary group is to be defined there is a substantial measure of agreement. Such a grouping is important in understanding capitalist societies they argue, and can be identified by the social relations of production. Each mode of production generates two fundamental classes, one exploiting class which is dominant politically and ideologically, and one exploited class, which is politically and ideologically dominated. A concrete society or social formation however 'involves more than two classes in so far as it is composed of various modes and forms of production. No social formation involves only two classes, but the two fundamental classes of any social formation are those of the dominant mode of production in that formation' (Poulantzas, 1975: 22). In a capitalist social formation then, the bourgeoisie and the proletariat constitute the two 'fundamental' classes, but others such as a middle class grouping are also found. Secondly, they stress an anti-voluntarist anti-distributive view of classes. Classes they argue are not 'things' but *relations*; they are composed not so much of individuals as of 'agents' in the production process, and exist only in the form of class struggles or class practices. Classes are thus defined in *relational* terms. Class struggle, as Wright (1980b: 212) indicates includes consciously organised conflicts between classes as well as 'conflicts which are directly implicated in the formation and transformation of classes, even if the combatants in the conflict are not strictly speaking class actors'. In this he draws on the distinction made by Przeworski (1977) that there is struggle both *between* classes and struggle *over* class.

The problem however with this approach, thus far at least, is the failure of the three writers to specify sufficiently the conditions for the autonomous operation of political and ideological elements. One writer who has attempted to overcome this problem in order to theoretically locate the notion of autonomy is Johnson (1977a, 1977b). He focuses on the processes of realisation and reproduction. The realisation process refers to the appropriation and accumulation of value;

surplus value in the capitalist mode of production, to the owners of the means of production—that is, to capital. This process under monopoly capital is transformed into a labour process Johnson (1977a) argues, based upon elaborate mechanisms of control in the form of bookkeeping, auditing and accountacy functions. The agents who carry out this function can be identified as new middle class as they express both a capital function (realisation) and a labour function (as part of an increasingly fragmented and routinised labour process). Doctors form part of this group on the basis of their reproduction of necessary labour power (simply keeping people at work).

Johnson's work directs attention towards the concept of reproduction which he argues occurs in all spheres, economic, political and ideological 'In the processes of the reproduction of labour power both the "professions" and the state play a major role, in health and education services and in the institutionalisation of knowledge including science and technology' (Johnson, 1977b: 228).

Johnson goes on to argue that historically the major trend in the reproduction of labour power has been the growing involvement of the state. This is related to the concentration of capital in the stage of monopoly capitalism, the consequent need for a mobile and transferrable labour force and the inability of other enterprises to fulfil this function (Johnson, 1977b: 228). The reproduction of labour power provides the theoretical basis for the autonomy of medicine; hence the role of the professional association in being able to structure and organise a part of the labour process—into a system of domination and subordination. Its success in other words, is not only to be located in terms of collective social mobility as the Parrys have done, but also 'because within the differentiated process of realisation it incorporates these specific powers within a secular organisational form' (Johnson, 1977b: 221).

Autonomy furthermore is based upon the process of occupationally generated definitions of professional service ('health', 'justice') becoming 'official' ones. Such a process however is historically specific Johnson (1977b: 229) argues:

For example the institutionalisation of 'colleague' control in medicine took place in the nineteenth century when social conditions associated with the rise of 'private' capitalism were conducive to 'professionalism' and occupational definitions of client need. In this field the existence of occupational power has, in the twentieth century been a limitation to state heteronomy and it has been the role of the state in the process of reproduction to underwrite existing occupationally generated definitions except where they conflict with the extension of health services to a clientele defined on the basis of citizenship.

The advantage of Johnson's analysis however is that it redirects the theoretical thrust of the earlier theorists towards a closer examination of the processes of reproduction. In this way he is able to locate theoretically the notion of autonomy and as well begin to locate the state patronage on which medical dominance is based. The medical profession gains state patronage through being 'allowed' a monopoly of occupationally generated definitions of service, in so far as these coincide with official definitions. This is what is meant when we speak of medicine as an important institution of social control; important in the reproduction of labour power. Medicine in other words mediates the relation between individuals and their bodies, and the state. However medicine is not only a mechanism of reproduction but also a beneficiary. The major benefit, which flows from its alliance with the dominant class, for my purposes here is medical dominance.

This discussion of autonomy however is incomplete without an analysis of professionalism, here viewed as an occupational ideology which legitimates autonomy for the doctors themselves. As Freidson (1970a: 80) argues, it is 'a deliberate rhetoric in the political process of lobbying, public relations and other forms of persuasion to attain a desirable end, full control over its work'. It is thus part of the dynamic of differentiation in the division of labour.

The ideology of professionalism however has wider ramifications reproducing aspects of the dominant ideology and thus promoting ideological hegemony which, as Gramsci (1971) argues, provides the basis for bourgeois rule in monopoly capitalism. In particular, professionalism reproduces what Habermas (1970) calls 'the ideology of expertise', the emphasis on technological rationality, on the claim to effectiveness, on individualism all of which lead to the claim that 'knowledge is beneficent power' yet legitimates inequality and elitism, as Larson (1977: 221–243) has shown for a number of capitalist countries. Now this is not to argue that ideology operates in a straightforward even way, but in a complex, contradictory and uneven fashion. The ideology of professionalism for instance is not reactionary in all situations but may be potentially subversive, so that it is an oversimplification to see the ideology of professionalism just as a microcosm of bourgeois ideology.

Extending the Gramscian analysis then, doctors must be seen as organic intellectuals which emerge in association with a new dominant class in advanced capitalism 'exercising the subaltern functions of social hegemony and political government' (Gramsci, 1971: 12). They are what Merrington (1968: 154) calls 'experts in legitimation'. They rationalise and provide a justification for the nature of that society, and thus 'act as the mediators of the realities of capitalism into values' (Davidson, 1968: 45). On this point it should be noted there is a striking parallel with some of the conservative medical sociological literature such as Parsons' which argues that medicine mediates important social values. The important difference is that for Gramsci these values serve class interests, tied as they are in the last analysis to the mode of production.

Authority and gender relations

The second level at which medical dominance is sustained is over the work of other health occupations. This level can be represented by the concept of authority. Here it is argued that to locate authority in theoretical terms involves considering both class and gender elements, and the relationship between them.

Doctors can be located as new middle class (under monopoly capitalism) irrespective of their nominal status as self-employed or salaried. Political and ideological factors 'over-determine' economic factors in locating them as an occupational group; in particular their role in the reproduction of labour power is important. Following Wright, Poulantzas' usage of the productive/unproductive dimension as determinant of class location is rejected. At the political and ideological level autonomy also locates doctors and some other health occupations such as optometrists, chiropractors, dentists etc as new middle class. It is still possible to identify these occupations as class groupings (against Wright) because what he describes as their contradictory location serves to give them a specific unity. Other health occupations however which are hierarchically subordinated to doctors within the medical division of labour have little or no autonomy in the performance of their work and are to be located as proletarian irrespective of their nominal productiveness or unproductiveness.

In so far as the occupational division of labour in health care has evolved through class struggle this has been both inter-and intra-class struggle. Hence the struggle between doctors and occupations such as optometrists, which exist outside medicine's formal control but are 'limited' in their institutionally defined area of expertise, is an intra-class struggle of authority rather than power (following Poulantzas). The struggle between doctors and 'subordinated' occupations is an inter-class struggle however; in other words one of power between classes and over class.

Yet authority relations cannot be analysed only in relation to class. Also located in the social relations of production is gender, a factor important to the analysis made here. A number of writers (eg Connell, 1979c; Sumner, 1979) have pointed to the lack of an adequate conceptualisation of gender relations and the sexual division of labour within many areas of sociology. As a recent writer on the professions has commented: 'theorists of professions ignore the fact that groups which have successfully professionalised have usually been male in composition' (Versluysen, 1981: 22).

The penetration of feminist writings into sociology and the gradual and overdue development of an awareness of the importance of gender as a source of social differentiation and inequality has led to a lively debate about the relative importance of class versus gender as dimensions of inequality—most explicit in Marxist-feminist literature (eg Kuhn and Wolpe, 1978; Barrett, 1980). The argument has been whether sexual divisions are ultimately reducible to the theory of class relations in capitalist society, or whether it is a structural element which is independent of class divisions though relevant to them.

The focus is upon the sexual division of labour, in capitalist societies defined as patriarchal, and here denoting an authority relation between the sexes involving male dominance. Many explanations view this division of labour as biologically based, a 'natural' division, springing from differences in reproductive functions. Such 'naturalism' I would argue (following Gamarnikow, 1978: 98) is ideological and the sexual division of labour must locate the relations between the sexes as social rather than biological categories. 'Naturalism' does not constitute an adequate explanation for the sexual division of labour in general or more specifically in health care. Sexual divisions therefore can be located within the social relations of production along with class divisions. These relations of production take their character from the capitalist mode of production and divide the 'agents' of production in different ways, including class and gender. Gender however has its own autonomous field, its own ideologies and own determinants. Gender relations take their specific character from their location in capitalist production relations. As a result not all struggles can be reduced to class struggles; some are gender struggles while others are over status. Gender and other struggles however have important implications for class struggle at the ideological level and constitute a part of the struggle *over* class which Przeworski (1977) details. In other words gender and other struggles become articulated with class struggles. Exactly how this occurs and the relative importance of class and gender vary with historical contingency. As Barrett (1980: 253) argues, the question of the relative importance of class and gender issues must be resolved historically rather than theoretically. In this study the historical context in which this debate is analysed, as it affected the development of the division of labour, is the struggle between midwives and general practitioners/obstetricians. This struggle had both gender and class dimensions.

Medical sovereignty and professionalism

The third level at which medical dominance is sustained is in the wider societal arena. The consequence of state patronage of medicine is that members of the occupation have become institutionalised experts on all matters related to health. This third level is designated as medical sovereignty.

Professional dominance for Freidson (1970a), what I have called medical dominance, has a dual foundation. One of these is the esoteric knowledge which the occupation holds, the other the patronage of the state. While he correctly identifies the internal cognitive structures which constitute medical knowledge as crucial to the establishment of medical dominance, he does not proceed to analyse theoretically the relationship between these two foundations; in short, how much does the sort of knowledge used by medicine in its practice account for the patronage of medicine by the capitalist state? In order to do this, it is necessary to examine the notion of 'compatibility' or 'constellation of interests' between the knowledge utilised in medical practice and class interests. These interests which have been pointed to but not analysed by other writers such as Berlant are represented both within the health arena, and the wider society.

In order to do this, it is necessary firstly to examine medical know-ledge itself, in particular what has come to be called 'scientific medicine', defined here as the field of clinical practice carried out by graduates of training institutions which teach the scientific, clinical and research orientations of the occupational association known as the Australian Medical Association. The debate about what constitutes knowledge, science and its relationship to ideology is a highly contentious one. The position adopted here follows that of Rose and Rose (1977: 13) who argue that both 'terrains' exist; there is science and there is ideology but there is a constant battle between the two, with ideology frequently masquerading as science. Technology is the commodity form of knowledge, developed to be consistent with capitalist production relations, and 'scientised' (ie brought into a close relationship with science) in the late nineteenth century (see Habermas, 1970). Importantly, technology may be penetrated by ideological elements in the same way as sicence.

Applied to the medical arena, my argument is that scientific medicine, particularly clinical medicine, is an amalgam of different types of knowledge, particularly science and ideology. Clinical medicine is the actual practice of medicine as an occupational group and may be contrasted with 'experimental medicine' which is carried on in a laboratory. Together they constitute scientific medicine. Medical technology can likewise be seen as the commodity form of medical knowledge.

In what ways then is clinical medicine ideological? As a first response, it is quite easy to demonstrate that clinical medicine utilises types of knowledge other than science. Elements of magical thinking have been demonstrated in the practice of clinical medicine for example (Roth, 1957). To be completely scientific, decisions would be made solely on the grounds of the theoretical basis of clinical practice (ie anatomy, physiology etc)—what might be called 'textbook knowledge'. A number of researchers have found that knowledge from the doctor's own experience was also important in medical decision making and at times was considered superior to 'textbook knowledge' (eg Freidson, 1970a). At times Freidson found, arguments based on the doctor's own clinical experience (a type of empiricism), could only be countered by arguments based upon greater clinical experience. This is given recognition with the stress still found on clinical medicine being an 'art' as well as a 'science'; in other words other types of knowledge are also the basis for decision making and actual practice. Following from the view of ideology adopted as having a material reality, all of the actions which constitute clinical practice may also be ideological practices and operate at a micro level (such as the doctor-patient relationship) to maintain and reproduce macrostructures, the capitalist mode of production. The 'laying on of hands' (ie *examining* patients), *communicating* with patients and *writing* prescriptions and certificates may all have ideological elements or effects. Medical certificates for example are required to legitimise a patient's absence from work. By the doctor's control over such certificates he or she is in a position to 'enforce industrial or home discipline through ideological messages about the work ethic or by denying the patient certification for illness' (Waterman and Waitzkin, 1977: 50).

Yet the task of specifying exactly which aspects of medical practice are scientific and what are ideological is a difficult one, since while the two are analytically distinct they are variably fused in practice. Something scientific such as the prescription of pills to alleviate medical conditions, for instance, may have ideological effects since its effect may be to individualise that patient's problem rather than to examine the social and political conditions which gave rise to it. Valium for example *does* act as a muscle relaxant (ie has a scientific basis) but may have an ideological effect to individualise a social and political problem resulting from a patriarchal division of labour ('suburban neurosis'). By the same token an ideology may be built on a sicentific basis.

The position adopted here is that the principal question is the political one. How did certain sorts of knowledge gain class and state patronage so as to permit the holders of that knowledge to achieve a position of dominance? To answer this question involves analysis of the process of legitimation. How scientific knowledge becomes legitimated illustrates the fusion of scientific and ideological (social and political) elements.

The emphasis of legitimation of, for example, different bodies of knowledge and practices such as medicine and chiropractic, avoids the thorny issue outlined by Habermas (1976) of whether one body of knowledge has greater 'truth value' than the other. Legitimacy is not related to a single 'truth' standard, even if such a standard could be decided on the basis of criteria other than those internal to the body of knowledge itself. What is important is that legitimacy is a process whereby a set of practices is accepted as authoritative and becomes hegemonic. This process involves the political process of justification. In modern capitalist societies such justification is strongly based on the idea of 'science as truth' and on the notion of effectiveness. In the claim for legitimacy, scientific medicine drew on both of these. However while there were elements of genuine scientific advance which should not be underrated, the claimed effects of these changes by medicine have been overstated (see Powles, 1973). Nonetheless the claim to effectiveness became an important component of the ideology of medicine and one utilised politically to legitimate medical dominance.

Thus the process of legitimation of scientific medicine is important to this study as is its effect on the evolution of the occupational division of labour. The process, following Kuhn (1970), must be seen as as much a social and political one as a technical or scientific one.

Most of the conventional positivistic accounts of the development of medical history have a Popperian theoretical basis. According to these accounts 'scientific medicine' is seen as the result of a relatively unproblematic combination of science on one hand and medicine on the other, in the nineteenth century. Medical knowledge accumulates on a trial-and-error basis, so meeting the criterion of falsification stressed by Popper (1959). As a number of writers have pointed out however (eg Figlio, 1977) these accounts ignore the social and economic origins of scientific medicine, and also tend to gloss over the political and social struggles involved in the establishment of scientific medicine over its competitors in the health field.

To do justice to the complex social and political process by which scientific medicine developed requires an analysis along Kuhnian lines of discontinuities in the growth process of knowledge formation through paradigms and scientific revolutions (Kuhn, 1970). Such transformations involves social and political action, including (against Kuhn) class action. On this basis I would argue that development of medical knowledge is not so much one of evolution and transition from 'prescientific' to 'scientific medicine' but one of discontinuity and transformation between different paradigms of medical knowledge from what I shall call the *Individualist* mode of medical production to the *Corporatist* mode. In other words there was a qualitative difference between the knowledge upon which scientific medical practice was based and that of prescientific medicine. Over the last decade of the nineteenth century and first decades of the twentieth century there was a change in paradigms with at least some major elements of incommensurability between the two. What is particularly relevant for our purposes here is that the different paradigms result in a different social organisation of health care and that understanding the change is crucial to explaining the notion of 'medical dominance'.

The Individualist mode, symbolised by the doctor's black bag was based on a relatively simple technology most of which could be carried in such a bag. Most medical care was provided at home, at the patient's bedside. Medical records tended to be uncodified; that is to say carried around in the doctor's head rather than written down. Medical care as a commodity was thus 'produced' on a small scale, by small scale petit bourgeois producer professionals. It was labour intensive with a stress on the classification of disease. The Corporatist mode by contrast must be viewed as a qualitatively different approach to medicine, more appropriately symbolised by the pathology laboratory. It is capital intensive, centralised in the hospital which became organised on factory-like lines, involving capitalist production methods in practice and research including codified or written down records, an emphasis on symptomatology and universal drugs. Armstrong (1979) has characterised the key difference as being in the source of medical knowledge from 'clinical sense' to 'clinical science'. Also of particular relevance for present purposes it involved factory-like hierarchies of workers, greater specialisation and the emergence of a complex division of labour. The Corporatist mode also required a much greater schooling base; thus stratifying medicine along class and gender lines much more than the Individualist mode.

Such an interpretation of the development of medical knowledge differs considerably from most accounts of nineteenth century medicine which stress the differences between the various sects, such as allopathy and homeopathy. From the perspective given above however it is argued that both represented the same Individualist mode of production. The debate between them, as observers such as Rothstein (1972) have pointed out, was mainly on the relative effectiveness rather than their theoretical incompatibility. The differences between allopathy and homeopathy can be seen mainly as marketing differences; one gave large amounts of drugs and bled the patient profusely, the other gave minimal drugs and didn't bleed. Both were petit bourgeois professionals working in medicine at the expense of lay healers such as 'quacks' and midwives who were overwhelmingly working class. The Corporatists mode on the other hand represented a different paradigm, so that allopathy did not just evolve into scientific medicine as is usually claimed. Most of the practioners who took up scientific medicine, as Berliner (pers. comm.) has argued, were originally allopaths but they did not just use the name scientific for the legitimacy it gave. Rather what we call 'scientific' medicine (which I have argued involves an amalgam of scientific and ideological elements) implies a qualitatively different mode of medical production leading to a transition from individual entrepreneurs to corporate capital. Homeopathy also eventually (though later) largely abandoned the Individualist mode and became involved in the Corporatist mode.

Now this should not be taken to mean that the change in paradigms had the nature of a sudden rupture over a short period of time, nor that it was even. Clinical evidence (ie from personal experience) is still important in medical decision-making as Freidson (1970a) has shown. Nor is it to argue that the modern general practitioner is merely a survival from the Individualist mode. General practice itself has been transformed by integration into pathology services, decline in home visits etc, all of which reflect processes internal to industrial capitalism. The point is that the emergence of the Corporatist mode, it can be argued, has its basis in a specific type of medical knowledge (germ theory). Much of the continuing success of medicine further-more can be attributed to the ability to articulate germ theory to other types of knowledge such as chemotherapy. But the process by which the Corporatist mode became accepted and predominant is indis-solubly scientific and also political.

The scientific element was provided by the actions and discoveries of doctors and medical researches themselves. Major discoveries such as those of Pasteur and Koch resulted in a change in medical practice towards more 'scientific medicine'. Yet while they were important they provide a less than adequate explanation of why the transition took place. In particular they underemphasise the importance of the social process of their implementation. Furthermore as Jamous and Peloille (1970: 117) have shown recognition needs to be made of the way in which the knowledge base of an occupation, as part of its occu-pational ideology, can be shaped so as to serve the needs of the practi-tioners. In particular they show how indeterminate aspects of medical practice can be stressed as a defence against outside evaluation and protection of autonomy.

To explore the political aspects of the process by which the Cor-poratist mode became accepted requires an analysis of the issue of compatibility between the type of medical knowledge generated and the perceived interest of the dominant class in the social formation. The compatibility issue has been explored at length by other writers mainly in the American context (especially Berliner, 1977; Renaud, 1977; Brown, 1979). The Corporatist mode of medical production entailed a view of disease as being the result of germs; that is specific causative agents. Disease was thus an individual and biological pheno-menon rather than a social and political one. In crude terms then it was 'germs that made people sick' rather than 'capitalism making people sick'. Such emphasis thus diverted attention away from the social and structural causation of disease. The dominant class also supported the new mode because of the claims by doctors that it would result in a healthier workforce; thus ensuring greater productivity and a more stable society. It also contributed significantly to the creation and maintenance of ideological hegemony in formulating a new culture appropriate to and supportive of industrial capitalism. The industrial analogy of the body as a machine for instance with replaceable parts and 'engineering solutions' was a feature of this.

With its aparent neutrality, the new paradigm of scientific medicine had considerable ideological and cultural advantages for the ruling class. This was particularly, so Brown (1976) argues, in the realm of imperialism where medical relief replaced missionaries as the penetrating arm of capitalism. The new paradigm however, while apparently neutral, was penetrated by ideological elements supportive of the interests of the dominant class. Three are particularly relevant here. Firstly the Corporatist mode raises some questions about for instance the causation of disease (at a simple level, what 'germ' caused this disease?) and not others (how are the effects of these germs mediated through the social and environmental milieu?). An example would be the search for the 'cause' of cancer in specific aetiological agents such as viruses. Such an approach has dominated cancer research and only recently is the recognition growing of the importance of environmental factors conditioned by economic and social forces (Chubin and Studer, 1978). Secondly this paradigm has ideological effects in proposing individualist solutions to what are structural problems. C Wright Mills (1956) has shown how this is a general feature of ideology in capitalist societies. The valium example noted previously exemplifies this. Thirdly, the Corporatist mode of medical production is ideological in its promotion of the 'ideology of expertise'. Only those who have 'expert knowledge' are competent to judge in health issues in this case, despite the ease of demonstrating within the literature that medical decisions are often made as much on social and moral grounds as on purely medical ones (eg Posner, 1977; Hughes, 1977). This ideology encourages a sense of apolitical passivity, of fatalism on the part of those who do not have this expertise as Swingewood (1975) has argued.

Certain types of medical knowledge in other words clearly served dominant class interests against dominated class interests. Although medical knowledge generated its own internal logic, its development was fostered by capital because of its compatibility with dominant class interests. This is not to argue mechanistically that it was controlled by 'capital', or even a 'tool' developed by medicine and the corporate class (as Brown, 1979 does). Knowledge is not passively reproduced by the economic structure; the forces and relations of production relate dialectically (see Mishra, 1979). Nor is it to argue for a functionalist type causality explained by the 'needs of capital' to maintain capitalism. Rather I am arguing for the sponsorship and support of the dominant class for the Corporatist mode of medical production in terms of its affinity with dominant class interests.

Thus the process has been of benefit to the powerful in society. What is of more interest for our purposes is to examine the benefits to doctors. The major one was that medicine gained the legitimacy of science itself. The discontinuity in medical knowledge took place against the background of the development of the capitalist mode of production from laissez-faire to monopoly capitalism. Several features of this process are relevant to the present discussion, the important one for present purposes being the rise of science as a new form of legitimacy in all areas of society. Science emerged as a form of legitimacy with the stress on the 'ideology of efficiency', Larson (1977) argues for the United States, but as Roe (1976) has shown was prevalent in Australia also. Medicine felt the impact of the new form of legitimation as did many other areas of society including agriculture, housework (domestic science), management, and many others. As Larson (1977: 137) argues, the structural transformation of the capitalist mode of production:

> corresponds to a shift in ideology toward new forms of legitimation of power. At the core the emergent conception of authority appeals to the rationality of science: science as a method and as a world view, more than as a body of knowledge—and to the rationality of scientifically oriented experts who act in the bureaucratised institutions of the new social order.

Medicine in other words gained a strategic advantage over other health occupations and one which secured for it a position of dominance. The Corporatist mode furthermore provided the basis for specialisation in the health division of labour. The mechanistic approach to understanding health and disease provided an internal logic for the development of scientific medicine and was reflected in specialisation in medical knowledge and practice that evolved around component parts of that body machine, ie cardiology, neurology etc (see Navarro, 1980: 199). The 'ideology of expertise' furthermore, taking its specific form in the human services arena as professionalism, and legitimates an hierarchical division of labour in which those who are the experts are the obvious controllers of that division of labour. Authority thus becomes equated with expertise as Peterson argues (1978: 286). Professionalism legitimates the health division of labour, it is the ideological representation of the manual/mental labour distinction within the health arena. As such it must be seen basically as associated with class and gender domination. It legitimates new middle class and a largely male domination of lucrative healing tasks and thus mystifies what is basically a class interest. As

Segall (1977) comments 'professionalism is an ideological justification for the purveyor of commodities based upon knowledge and skill to promote their economic and social interests in a market economy'. From this patronage the capitalist social order won important cultural and ideological advantages in the maintenance of bourgeois hegemony. Thus as Brown argues 'the knowledge generated by scientific medicine and the techniques of medical technology provided the basis for the physicians claim to a monopoly of authority over the practice of medicine' (Brown, 1979: 237).

This patronage is also relevant for the phenomenon of medical sovereignty. As aspect of ideological hegemony relevant for present purposes is the control of knowledges such as science. Medicine for instance is legitimated through science and has co-opted its legitimating powers so that an attack on medicine is usually seen as an attack on science itself. The phenomenon referred to as 'medicalisation' (eg by Illich, 1976), the extension of the medical paradigm into the so-called mental health field as psychiatry and thereby into morality and law, is a classic example of the extension of ideological hegemony.

Professions and the state

In this chapter so far I have analysed the theoretical foundations of autonomy, authority and medical sovereignty; the three levels at which medical dominance is sustained. Throughout the chapter I have been arguing that the development of the division of labour in health care which results in medical dominance, takes place against a politico-economic backdrop, which includes the activities of the capitalist state; analysis of which is indispensable to the study.

Most debate on the democratic capitalist state has concerned the relationship between state institutions and the dominant class. The position taken here is to argue for a degree of insulation of the state apparatus and the dominant class. The state, without acting as its direct representative, serves the interests of the dominant class in an overall though indirect sense of maintenance; of the economy, of political order and of legitimacy. It also resolves disputes between the fractions of the dominant class. It thus maintains the social fabric within the relations of production and in that way serves the political interests of the dominant class without being directly subordinate to that class (see O'Malley, 1979).

Following Poulantzas (1978: 128–9), the state is not a 'thing' but the material condensation of a balance of forces and relations. It is the site of class struggle and class relationships, both inter-class and intra-class, since one of the struggles therein is between different fractions of the ruling class. Rather than being a tool of the dominant class it must integrate all classes within the capitalist mode of production. From this point of view the state is a type of relationship within a material framework and organisation. This framework is constituted by an array of judicial, legislative, military and coercive institutions which together comprise the state bureaucracy of which the health bureaucracy is a part. The state gains its autonomy in part from the existence of this bureaucracy which develops its own interests and material conditions of existence, so at the day-to-day level bureaucratic officials manage the capitalist society. It is the relationship between the institutions within the framework which constitute the state. The relationship furthermore is one involving class and other struggles. These struggles 'have a specific presence within the structure of the State—a presence that is expressed by the State's material framework bound up with relations of production, by its hierarchical-bureaucratic organisation, and by the reproduction of the social division of labour within the State' (Poulantzas, 1978: 141).

The precise configuration of these state institutions (such as health), Poulantzas goes on to argue, will depend on the 'relationship of forces' and thus will vary historically to organise hegemony. To achieve this he argues, 'the State installs particularly the petty bourgeoisie ... as veritable props of the power bloc, dislocating their alliance with the working class. The resulting alliances-compromises and relationship of forces are embodied in the structure of the particular state apparatus that fulfills this function' (Poulantzas, 1978: 142).

Applied concretely to the health arena, such an alliance between new middle class doctors and the state is at the root of the phenomenon of medical dominance. Also we can distinguish between the bureaucracy (the health department) which may itself be penetrated by medical dominance, and with its own interests, as against the judiciary and legislature which may not necessarily be supportive of medical dominance but may reflect other class positions. As a result legislation may sometimes be supportive of medical dominance and other times not (for example passing statutory registration legislation for chiropractic). As a result, I am not implying that the relationship between doctors, the ruling class and the state (especially the legislative arm) has been an uneventful one. Indeed, some of the major political battles of the twentieth century (eg the 1949 nationalisation struggle and High Court challenge in Australia) have been fought between the state and medicine (see Hunter, 1969).

Viewing the state not as a unified omniscient force but as a set of relations made up of conflicting and competing groupings, renders the sphere of legislation which is important to the analysis here, a problematical one. Ideology and struggle within the legislative process means that legislation cannot be reduced only to the requirements of capital but that the sphere of concrete experience of individuals is also important. The state does not involve some sort of equilibrium or stable state. The struggle between classes, with the working class attempting to achieve the hegemony of its own ideology ensures that bourgeois ideological hegemony is at best uneven and incomplete.

Yet the autonomy of the state is only a partial one and the argument given should not be read as a return to interest group or power elite theory. The state gains its capitalist character from its primary role in supporting and defending the capitalist economy. As Habermas (1976) and O'Connor (1973) have shown there are two conflicting parts to this role: capital accumulation and legitimation. In other words the state must protect the economic interests of the dominant class without appearing to do so. This contradictory aspect of the state ensures its relative autonomy. To maintain the integration of all classes in the capitalist social formation necessary for legitimation, naked class domination is impossible. Hence the emphasis on the maintenance of ideological hegemony to which doctors contribute. The state intervenes to facilitate cultural reproduction in those areas of science and culture (such as medicine) which are consistent with the relations of production. Hence the state intervenes in the health arena in passing legislation, funding medical schools, providing research grants etc, all of which ensure this ideological reproduction.

The changing role of the capitalist state is important to this study. Such a development is related to the changing capitalist mode of production. The impetus of capital accumulation makes capitalism a particularly dynamic system, in an unplanned and autonomous way developing the productive forces, concentrating and centralising capital, dissolving previous modes of production, and establishing the world economic system. This development has been conceptualised through stages; capitalism has developed from a 'laissez-faire' stage of private, competitive capitalism to a stage of advanced, monopoly or corporate capitalism today. One consequence of this has already been analysed, the growth of science as a world view and source of legitimation penetrated by ideology. The other is the growth of state intervention. Now as Gough (1979) warns, the development of capitalism has been uneven and thus it is difficult to generalise across different countries. 'Laissez-faire' capitalism for instance took by far its most vigorous form in the United Kingdom and the settlement of Australia was an early outgrowth of the very early stages of the development of British capitalism.

Studies of the development of Australian capitalism are very thin on the ground, but certainly it appears that the 'laissez-faire' stage of capitalism in the sense of minimal state intervention never really existed in Australia (Wheelwright, 1976). The state was important in providing the conditions for capital accumulation right from the start (the use of convict labour to build a basic infrastructure) and in the provision of tariff barriers to encourage local industry. But while some of the reality of 'laissez-faire' was different, much of its attendant ideology is certainly found. 'Laissez-faire' itself refers to the desirability (if not the practicality) of state non-intervention in economic affairs. It was associated on the one hand with a belief in the moral desirability of maximum freedom for individuals (libertarianism), and on the other with 'liberalism', the belief in the desirability of maximising economic competition. The transition from laissez-faire to monopoly capitalism is difficult to locate temporally. Wheelwright (1976) uses post World War II as the dividing point but the question is far from settled. Certainly it must be seen as a fairly lengthy transition.

Given this politico-economic backdrop we are able to examine the nature of state intervention in the health sector. Such state intervention is aimed both at facilitating capital accumulation and legitimation. A means of analysing such state intervention in health is provided by Navarro (1976: 209–14). Drawing heavily on the work of Offe (1972), Navarro argues that state intervention is of two broad types. Negative selection mechanisms are modes of intervention which exclude those strategies which conflict with the class nature of capitalist society (for example a totally socialised health service). Positive selection mechanisms on the other hand generate and stimulate a positive response favourable to capital accumulation.

In the health arena the state is involved mainly in positive selection mechanisms in the form of licensing, particularly in the era of monopoly capitalism. Licensing is a form of legal protection for the occupational territories of various health occupations from competitors. The state in other words provides those occupations with statutory registration in the form of licensing laws as a means of self-defence against encroachment upon their means of livelihood. The struggle for licensing and over the content of the legislation by various occupations is a major process to be analysed in this thesis. Licensing provides the legal foundation for the division of labour and thereby medical dominance. The domination of medicine is sustained by the legal definition of the occupational territories of other health occupations. This is what is meant when we say medicine enjoys state patronage.

On this basis we can distinguish three phases in the development of relationships between medicine and the state. The first entails minimal state intervention and regulation of the health arena; rather the allocation of health resources was left to market forces with only limited and covert state patronage. This period lasted until about 1900. After this time the second phase began as the state began to intervene more actively in health matters. Initially, up until about the Second World War the state statutorily endorsed medicine's position of dominance, delegating responsibility for health matters to medicine and under-writing medicine's position. The third phase however, which might tentatively be located in the post World War II period, is characterised by less willingness of the state to so wholeheartedly endorse and patro-nise medicine, with conflict emerging and a rearguard action being fought by medicine to preserve its pre-eminent position. Other health occupations during this period would increasingly look to the state for legitimation through statutory registration rather than medicine itself. Formerly legitimation had been only achieved by the consent of medi-cine. This became less important during the third stage.

The complex nature of the relationship between medicine and the state is also seen in the frustration of the attempt by medicine to secure a monopoly by the need of the state to preserve its legitimation. In two ways has this been important to the historical analysis here, and a specific historical feature of Australian society. One is the issue of state parochialism. The political development of Australia as separate and competing states (Victoria, New South Wales, etc) until federa-tion in 1901 made the charge of 'lagging behind other states' in certain aspects a powerful stimulus to action, as we will see in the historical analysis to follow. The other issue was the rural/urban one. With the allocation of medical manpower left to market forces the rural/urban disparities which have always plagued Western capitalist countries, at times thwarted medicine in its attempt to control competition. In the interests of basic legitimacy the state at some times in Victoria's development refused to grant state patronage to that extent. Restrictions on practice by health workers other than doctors would in some rural areas have left nobody to provide health care. Both of these issues of legitimacy were influential in the development of the division of labour in health care in Victoria, as will be seen.

The division of labour

Having outlined the theoretical bases for autonomy, authority and medical sovereignty, the remaining task is to consider the division of labour itself as well as the major alternative explanation for its deve-lopment in the health arena.

There are several aspects of the division of labour in health care which need to be discussed. Firstly a distinction must be made between the informal unpaid health 'workers', mainly family members and volunteers (and usually women) and the formal paid occupationally based division of labour. As Davies (1979b: 518) has argued the place of these workers in the division of labour and the relationship between paid formal and unpaid informal elements remains largely untheo-rised and this study is no exception.

Secondly, drawing upon the insights derived from interactionism, a distinction must also be drawn (following Goldie, 1977) between the division of labour as a *negotiated* or *imposed* phenomenon. That negotiation in the allocation of tasks is possible and common, has been documented by a variety of researchers, in a number of institutional settings (see for example Goldie, 1977; Horobin and McIntosh, 1977). As Freidson (1976: 311) comments, the division of labour in health must be seen, at least partially as:

a process of social interaction in the course of which participants are continually engaged in attempting to define, establish, maintain and renew the tasks they perform and the relationships with others which their tasks presuppose ... (since) most of the time the limits to interaction posed by consensual conceptions of 'scientific' necessity and legal propriety are sufficiently broad and permissive that a variety of bargains is possible for the participants.

While acknowledging that negotiation is common, Freidson recognises that 'there are boundaires set on what will be considered legitimate to negotiate, how the negotiations will take place and what bargains can be struck'. My concern is with this *imposed* division of labour, the formal task differentiation, and how that has evolved. The two undoubtedly are related however; the everyday world of work, taken historically is one of the factors that has influenced the formal framework.

Thirdly the division of labour within health care in particular, has developed somewhat differently from its development generally within industry. In the industrial sphere the development of capitalism has resulted in the gradual substitution of capital for labour as the organic composition of capital ratio has increased. In other words, the division of labour in many industries has become more capital intensive and the demand for labour in most work processes has decreased. In health care however the development of the division of labour has generally been marked by increasing capital *and* labour intensiveness. Some technical developments can be designated as labour saving, for example an autoclave machine to sterilise instruments replaces the person who formerly boiled up the instruments themselves. Generally however the development of new medical technology has spawned the development of new occupations. For example the development of X-ray machines stimulated the development of two new health occupations, radiologists and radiographers, without this development displacing any other occupation.

The actual historical process of differentiation in the division of labour is a complex one and involves two distinct processes of specialisation. The first of these I have called *horizontal* specialisation and has occurred within particular occupations, especially medicine. The emergence of medical specialists as Rosen (1944) has argued, is the result of two complementary processes. One is segmentation in which a separate specialised field (ie occupying a distinct occupational territory), divides into two or more separate specialties. For example Eye, Ear, Nose and Throat specialists divided into ophthalmologists (interested in eyes) and ENT (Ear, Nose and Throat) specialists. The second process is accretion whereby a mutual field of interest overlapping two specialties leads to a merger of interests and the appearance of a new specialty relating specifically to that overlapping area. Paediatrics for example emerged from both specialist physicians (ie in internal medicine) and general practitioners interested in diseases of childhood.

The existence of (horizontal) specialisation within occupations has been important to the emergence of the division of labour in health care. This phenomenon, called segmentation by Bucher and Strauss (1961) has meant that at times health occupations have had difficulty acting collectively with the result that their political strength has been undermined. This has been particularly the case with the medical profession and its occupation association, the Australian Medical Association. Because of internal segmentation, Scotton (1974) argues that the AMA must be seen as more akin to a trade union congress than a single monolithic trade union (see also McGrath, 1975). Indeed, efforts on the part of occupational associations within the health arena to contain segmentation have been a major feature of the process examined here.

The second process of specialisation I have termed *vertical* specialisation. This process is more important to this study as it provides the bases for the hierarchicalisation of the health division of labour. The delimitation of occupational territory, which is the result of the historical process of differentiation in the division of labour (analysed here), has resulted in a complex hierarchy of health workers. How this vertical specialisation occurred is important to the subsequent analysis. Two complementary processes appear to operate, one involving subprofessional dominance, the other secondary deskilling (see Larkin, 1978, 1981). As Everett Hughes (1958) has argued, all occupations have a component of 'dirty work', the less pleasant, more mundane aspects of an occupation's work tasks. What has occurred has been the phenomenon of 'pass-the-task' by which these less pleasant, more routine, mundane tasks have been delegated to a subordinate occupation further down the hierarchy, often specifically created for the purpose of carrying out those tasks. Nursing is the classic example of this process called subprofessional dominance. The occupation of nursing was created historically to provide 'care', while doctors provide the 'cure'. Nurses carry out the more routine tasks associated with healing such as taking observations (temperature etc) (see Krause, 1977: 48–56). The process is reproduced over time, as evidenced by the fact that nursing has subsequently hived off some of its 'dirty work' to another health occupation; nursing aides.

The other process operating is secondary deskilling. By this process some health occupations are legally barred from performing certain tasks which constitute part of the occupational territory of medicine. Radiographers for example cannot legally interpret the X-rays they take, nor optometrists diagnose ocular pathology. Anaesthesiology was delegated to nursing by medicine, but when it was realised to be a potentially lucrative medical specialty, it was taken back into medical hands (Krause, 1977: 54). By these two processes the complex division of labour has emerged.

Opposing technological determinism

The major alternative explanation for the phenomenon of medical dominance can be termed a technological determinist one and is specifically argued against. According to this explanation, science and technology develop and determine an increasingly differentiated division of labour. Sax (1972), for instance, in his analysis of the Australian health care system argues that 'as technology becomes more sophisticated professions grow, specialisation occurs and new professions are born'. Technological imperatives provided by medical technology result in specialisation of occupation tasks and the development of new medical occupations as the health division becomes more differentiated. For example, when X-ray machines were invented, there was obviously a need for a new medical occupation—X-ray technician, to operate the new and improved technology. Such differentiation is a feature of the process of modernisation or industrialism assumed to be affecting all societies rather than a feature of capitalism per se. Such an approach is epitomised by the work of Illich (1976) and Mechanic (1976). Illich (1976: 211) for example argues that 'pathogenic medicine is the result of industrial overproduction' rather than being tied to the system of economic relationships in which people live. In other words the requirements of the new scientific, technological medicine, by imposing its own limits on the forms of social organisation possible, was thus the determining force in the development of modern health care. In particular it determined a complex division of labour which was aimed at efficiency; that is coping with the new developments such as X-ray machines in the most rational way.

Based upon the arguments made in this chapter, it is this technological determinist approach to understanding the development of health care and the health division of labour against which I specifically wish to argue. Firstly as a number of writers have argued it assumes 'technological rationality' which in capitalist societies is a form of ideology (Marcuse, 1971; Blackburn, 1969). Such an ideology mystifies the social relations upon which that technology is based and thus is a force in maintaining ideological hegemony in society. Mandel (1975: 59) argues that 'belief in the omnipotence of technology is the specific form of bourgeois ideology in late capitalism'. This ideology produces a technocratic approach to problems created in society; that is it proposes the ability to find technical solutions to health problems. This has resulted in an 'engineering' approach towards ill-health; people are made healthy by technological fixes in the form of replacement surgery or what the pharmaceutical companies refer to as 'wonder drugs'. Science and technology as Habermas (1970) argues, have become new forms of authority in capitalist societies and also new forms of domination.

Secondly, technological determinism conflates the technical division of labour (that is by occupation, on-the-job) with the social division of labour (that is in society as a whole by class, gender etc), so as to stress the primacy of the technical over the social. Contrary to this I have argued for the primacy of the social over the technical in the same way as the social relations of production determine the technical relations of production. Technology cannot be reified, it is not a 'thing' but a system of social relationships and thus technology itself must be separated from the social relationships which emerge to cope with that relationship. These relationships are a microcosm of the broader social structure which is stratified and divided along class and gender lines. To return to the X-ray machine example, to argue that the invention of such a machine created the necessity for operators (X-ray technicians) to be trained and organised into an occupation to operate that machinery does not explain why those technicians are disproportionately women, and work under the direction of the controllers of medical care, doctors, and at much lower payment rates. The latter factors result from the social division of labour in general, not from the technological imperatives of the new machines.

Technological determinism thus tends to ignore the interaction of society with technology; that is, the way in which technology and society shape each other dialectically. In capitalist societies labour is subservient to capital and it is capital that determines which technology is introduced and how that technology is utilised. It is the politico-economic organisation of society which generates certain types of technological innovation and ignores others. The introduction of new technology may generate new social forces such as an increasingly differentiated division of labour. But as Marglin (1974) has argued this division of labour is directed not so much at rationalisation and efficiency as the technological determinists argued, but at control and capital accumulation. In other words technical divisions in the labour process are determined by the relations of production in the production of surplus value (Braverman, 1974). Technological determinism in short is the ideological representation of the capitalist division of labour.

Applied more specifically to the health arena then, scientific medicine, with its technological emphasis, must be seen not as the determining force in the development of modern health care and particularly the division of labour associated with it. New technology was introduced into the health arena so as to strengthen rather than create the hierarchy of health occupations. Furthermore as I have argued specifically elsewhere (Willis, 1979) and examine generally here, hierarchy preceded technology. This is not to argue technological developments were inconsequential, indeed hierarchy and technology develop dialectically, that is in a mutually influencing way. But as Navarro (1976: 206) has argued in that dialectical relationship hierarchy has precedence. That hierarchy is based upon class and gender.

Indeed the emphasis on technological determinism and technological rationality can usefully be seen as an element of the ideology of medicine which legitimates medical dominance. To argue that the hierarchical division of labour which emerged from technological development was 'necessary' for coping with improvements in medical knowledge and techniques of practice, while it has powerful protective functions for medicine as Scull (1975: 221) has shown, ignores the complex social processes involved in the development of the division of labour, to be analysed here.

In other words what I am arguing is that given burgeoning medical technology in the health arena, this was appropriated by the occupational group with suitable class links and a compatible ideology. Its appropriation lead to state patronage which secured a position of dominance. Class and gender struggle have both been important to differentiation of the health division of labour.

3 The rise of medicine: the pre-scientific era

Medical dominance it has been argued, must be studied both historically and in terms of a struggle between various health occupations.
To explain medical dominance there are two 'moments' to be considered: its production and its reproduction. This chapter and the next
consider the first 'moment' of the production of medical dominance.
They examine how the division of labour in health care evolved such
that one occupation, medicine, gained a position of dominance in the
social structure of health care delivery. The historical process to be
analysed is the rise of medicine to a position of political and economic
power within the health arena.

The production of medical dominance can be analysed in two
stages. The first of these, considered in this chapter, is the development of medicine prior to the transition in paradigms. In conventional
medico-historical terms this might be called the 'pre-scientific era'.
The specific location chosen to examine this process historically is the
state of Victoria, Australia, beginning with the origins of settlement in
the 1830s. The development of medicine in Victoria is analysed until
about 1880, by which time the impact of scientific medicine and the
effects of the incorporation of earlier scientific discoveries into clinical
practice were on the way to being established.

The origins of the Victorian medical profession

The first non-Aboriginal medical practitioners to arrive in Australia
came with the first fleet in 1788, when the unwilling band of
'colonists' who were dropped on the shores of Port Jackson included
four naval surgeons who had been appointed to the civil establishment, a surgeon's mate (apprentice) and a convict 'bred to surgery'
(Dewdney, 1972: 269). The first non-Aboriginal practitioner to settle
permanently in the state of Victoria was Dr Barry Cotter in 1835,
although he came from Van Dieman's Land (Tasmania) not as a
medical practitioner, but in the role of manager in the grandiose
scheme of the Port Phillip Association of which Batman the 'founder'
of Melbourne had been the advance agent. The scheme had provision

for a medical officer and Dr Alexander Thomson arrived in March 1836 to fulfil that capacity. The hopes of the Port Phillip Association were dashed by the Colonial Office's refusal to recognise it however, and Lonsdale was sent from Sydney to administer the settlement. Thomson soon abandoned his medical post for the greener pastures of squatting and Cotter, with no estate to manage, reverted to practising medicine until 1837 when Dr Patrick Cussen, a military surgeon, arrived to take the post of 'Colonial Assistant Surgeon' and Cotter became the colony's first private medical practitioner. By 1841, when assisted immigration was underway to the colony, Melbourne listed eighteen physicians and surgeons among its more than 20,000 inhabitants (McKay, 1936: 421–422).

In this early period of development until the discovery of gold in the 1850s, the population increased gradually, being boosted by the regular arrival of immigrant ships from the United Kingdom. The ships brought medical men, along with others keen to try their hands at healing. Without any form of regulation except for official posts (such as coroner) there were no restrictions on the practice of medicine. In order to know something about who these early practitioners were, both qualified and unqualified, it is necessary to consider conditions in the United Kingdom.

The task of understanding the conditions of British life for medical practitioners in the mid-Victorian era (1858–1886) is made considerably easier by the recent work of Peterson (1978) entitled *The Medical Profession in Mid Victorian England*. The focus of this study it should be pointed out is a somewhat narrow one, both geographically, in examining only the London area and also conceptually in not relating developments to their wider social, political and economic context. Despite this limitation the work is a very useful detailed sociological history of medicine of the period. It is corroborated by other studies (eg Berlant, 1975; Parry and Parry, 1976) and provides insight into the reasons some medical practitioners chose to emigrate to Australia.

Peterson argues that it was impossible to talk of the medical profession at all before the Medical Act of 1858, and then of dubious value for a considerable time after that. Medical care was organised in a hierarchical social structure of three distinctly organised, legally defined status groups practising 'the *profession* of physic', 'the *craft* of surgery', and 'the apothecary's *trade*' (Peterson, 1978: 12, emphasis added).

The physicians were the highest status group, having university degrees and operating under a charter dating from 1518. Within this numerically small group (less than 5 per cent of all practitioners in 1847), there was an elite group who had attended Oxford or Cambridge and were thereby eligible for Fellowships of the College of Physicians. Surgery, the middle order of practitioner, was considered more of a craft. Historically surgery had been associated with Barbers until it became independent in 1745. Rather than being trained in a university, surgeons were trained by the apprenticeship system. Apothecaries constituted the bottom tier of the hierarchy and were linked historically with trade, having been part of the Grocers' Company until 1617. During the seventeenth and eighteenth centuries, apothecaries gradually expanded their occupational territory. Initially they had just dispensed drugs, gradually however they began to provide medical advice also. This extension of tasks was facilitated by the class orientation of the physicians, who saw themselves as providing just for the wealthy. As a result, the task of providing care for the bulk of the population fell to the lower order of practitioner, especially the apothecary, whose inexpensiveness secured him a practice. The right to provide what we now call primary medical care was legitimated by the Apothecaries Act of 1815.

These three orders constituted an occupational division of labour and as well reflected a 'preindustrial form of social structure and stratification' (Peterson, 1978: 12). The boundaries between the occupational territories of physicians and other practitioners was legally maintained by the charter of the Royal College of Physicians, which forbade the physician from practising surgery or from compounding his own drugs as an apothecary. However no such restrictions existed for surgeons and apothecaries and it become increasingly common during the nineteenth century for practitioners to hold joint qualifications as surgeon-apothecary (the early general practitioner).

The 1858 act unified these three groups into a single occupation under one central governing body. But although it can be seen as a victory for middle class interests against entrenched aristocratic privilege (Larson, 1977: 24), it did not remove the class differences between them. In fact Peterson argues, the differences were further accentuated by the development during the nineteenth century of the hospital as the centre of medical education. The development of the 'consultant', as an occupational group holding hospital or medical school appointments, became a further source of stratification within the occupation of medicine. Although there was occupational unity in the sense that all three orders became united into one occupation; the segmentation remained. During the nineteenth century, the corporate distinction between physicians, surgeons and apothecaries was gradually replaced as the major source of stratification by a distinction between the elite of the profession and the rank-and-file group. The elite consultant group was drawn largely from the leadership of the colleges in London, while on the other hand, the rank-and-file gradually became more homogenous. In Scotland, the situation was a little different in that universities offered joint qualifications in physic and surgery so that the occupational division of labour was less rigid.

Peterson argues that one of the major problems faced by medicine was the lack of effective medical knowledge. Those who were able to, such as physicians, drew more upon traditional class mechanisms to establish trust and as a source of status and prestige, so that 'the demonstrable efficacy of medical practice was not the source of the profession's prestige and authority, any more than the status of the Anglican clergy derived from the demonstrable effectiveness of prayer and ritual' (Peterson, 1978: 4). A 'scientific' mind was less important for the individual practitioner in establishing a career, than family connections, tact, grooming, manners and so on (Parry and Parry, 1976; Peterson, 1978; Stevens, 1966). The rudimentary state of medical knowledge Peterson argues, meant a lack of public confidence in doctors, so they tended to put their faith in these social criteria, or even preferred to consult an unlicensed practitioner.

Furthermore, because it was a cheaper form of training, the possibility of apprentice training meant that wider (middle class) recruitment was possible. Public school education for example was not important except for physicians. Peterson (1978: 201) argues that recruitment came especially from the rising capitalist class and in comparative status terms, medicine ranked lower than either army officers or high clergy such a bishops. The bulk of the profession in other words were unable to draw upon the social bases of prestige which were available to physicians, and their status suffered as a result (Parry and Parry, 1976). In opposing medical reform, the physicians expressed the social differences between them and the bulk of the profession. '[They are] imperfectly educated, all engaged in the trading, money making parts of the profession and not one in a hundred of them distinguished by anything like science or liberality of mind!' (Keetley, quoted in Peterson, 1978: 33).

Peterson argues that the rank-and-file medical practitioner was thus faced with low income, poor status and lack of cohesion. Under such conditions, establishing a practice was a formidable problem for many. Once qualified, a clientele had to be attracted in the face of considerable competition from both qualified and unqualified practitioners. This had to be achieved in the face of an oversupply of doctors (as in all professions, O'Boyle, 1970). The oversupply was a result, Musgrove (1959) argues, of the expansion of middle class education after 1830, which was not matched by a similar rate of expansion of middle class employment opportunities. Furthermore, unqualified practitioners of various types abounded. The elite of the occupation, the leaders of the corporations were largely untroubled by this competition as it had little effect on their practices, prestige and power. The rank-and-file of general practitioners however were very much in competition and much of the pressure for legislative restriction on unqualified practitioners came from them.

In an age when social appearances were more important than skill, the cost of setting up practice in a suitable manner was also expensive (see for instance Doyal, 1887). Once set up, the young practitioner could also look forward to some lean years. As Peterson (1978: 221) comments:

> it is possible to suggest that most medical men, more particularly the rank and file of G.P.'s were attempting to live as 'professional gentlement' on incomes that were at best marginal and most often below the income of £700 defined by the banks as required in order to sustain the paraphenalia of gentility.

The responses to these difficult conditions varied. One was the growth of medical specialisms as a form of medical entrepreneurship. This phenomenon Peterson (1978: 248–74) argues, was more related to economic survival and ambition that to technical innovation and the desire to do research. Faced with difficulty in establishing oneself in a general medical practice, one response was to concentrate only upon certain diseases or certain parts of the body and thereby attempt to build a reputation.

In such an overcrowded profession, the possibility of migration existed as a kind of safety valve for those practitioners unable to establish themselves in private practice.

> ... they could find no post likely to lead to settled practice in a town and rather than continue with their inability to attach themselves to a network of professional patronage, they left the country, some temporarily, some permanently. ... One can trace their progress from London to one, two or three provincial towns, perhaps back to London then a sea voyage, only to return to try again. For many the last resort was to emigration. Without connections in England they went to the colonies, frequently to Australia. In the colonial situation a man was on a more equal footing with his medical competitors. Social ties in these places were broken for all of them, and for their patients as well and few could enjoy the advantage of connection at the start. Prospects were thought to be good in colonial practice but the price was high. Personal values of family, friendship and home were sacrificed for the sake of a career. (Peterson, 1978: 124–126)

Unsuccessful career starters in the United Kingdom thus provided one group of emigrant doctors. Others undoubtedly came with considerable capital as indicated by the number who became established squatters (McKay 1936). The prospect of better opportunities in Australia, particularly the lure of gold in the 1850s encouraged many to emigrate while others came for medical reasons seeking relief from psithsis (such as tuberculosis) in the warmer climate (Inglis, 1958: 32).

The earliest demographic data on those who migrated to Victoria, is the Medical Registrar of 1863, provision for which had been incorporated in the first Medical Registration Act of 1862. This act established a medical register on which qualified practitioners could place their qualifications, and provides a reasonable indication of who migrated to Victoria. Three items of demographic information can be gained from the register. Firstly it demonstrates that most of the 527 practitioners on the register had qualified in England (43 per cent) while only six per cent had qualified outside the United Kingdom and Ireland. Secondly surgeons and surgeon-apothecaries predominated (60 per cent). There were relatively few practitioners qualified solely as physicians (four per cent) and in particular a notable absence of graduates from the prestigious Oxford or Cambridge medical schools. The first *Cyclopedia of Victoria* (Smith, 1903) which contained biographical details of the 'leading; citizens of the time, revealed only one medical practitioner, (W Balls-Headley) out of 70 listed, who had an Oxbridge training, (though entries were self-selecting). This evidence however does provide some support for the argument made by Peterson and also by O'Boyle (1970: 480) that Australia provided a safety-value for those who had 'failed to make the grade in English society'. Thirdly as would be expected it was mainly men in the early to mid-careers who emigrated.

Some information on those qualified practitioners who migrated to Australia is thus available. Less is available however concerning the unqualified ones. Certainly there were a sizeable number of Chinese doctors; in the census of 1861 they were counted together with Aboriginal practitioners, together numbering 61 (listed separately from the 592 physicians, surgeons, apothecaries, oculises and dentists) (Medical Record, 7.7.1863: 592). Others to arrive according to Gandevia (1971: 51), included a number who had been medical students at one time, a significant group of homeopathic practitioners as well as a considerable number without any qualifications but an interest at trying their hand at the art of healing.

The conditions of practice in early Victoria which influenced the development of the occupation, mirror those general historical processes which historians (such as Blainey, 1966) have pointed to as influencing the development of Victoria in general. The experiences of practitioners migrating to Victoria were many and various. A number became pastoralists and gave up their medical practices altogether. McKay (1936: 422) cites more than 40 practitioners who held pastoral leases at the time of the administrative separation of Victoria from NSW in 1851. It is likely that most of these would have arrived in Victoria with some capital in order to get established and squatters rapidly became the dominant class in Victoria.

A considerable number of doctors went to the goldfields after the discovery of gold in 1854, either following their patients as they left towns en masse, or to do some prospecting themselves, or, more commonly to combine both (Bowden, 1974). Competition on the goldfields was great, both between qualified practitioners and also between qualified and unqualified practitioners. Others combined the practice of medicine with other pursuits. The wine-making industry for example owes much to early medical practitioners who practised viticulture as a hobby. The names of Lindeman and Penfold are two that remain today.

However not all practitioners met with success. There are case histories of high mobility around Victoria as well as interstate and back to Britain in search of a stable and successful practice. One such case of high mobility is that of Dr George Wakefield who qualified as an apothecary in London in 1841, practised in four different locations in England before coming to Victoria where he practised at both Ballarat and Kerang, and planned a move to Collins St in the city just before his death in 1883 (LTL MS6331). There were also bankruptcies of doctors reported. Bowden (1974: 145) for instance reports the case of a medical practitioner who failed to make a satisfactory living despite two years on the goldfields. The difficulty in establishing a stable medical career, having been the original motivation for migrating to Australia, sometimes continued after arrival.

The age of controversy

This early period in the development of medical care in Victoria was dominated by controversies over appropriate treatments, both between qualified medical practitioners (ie those with some recognised training), and also between qualified and unqualified practitioners of various types. These controversies resulted from the state of medical knowledge of the time, in particular the lack of what Larson (1977) calls 'a secure cognitive basis' for medicine. The rudimentary knowledge of disease and an inability to demonstrate effectiveness of treatments meant that the practice of medicine could not be based on a unified, standardised knowledge base as was possible later. Yet the universality of need for medical services on the part of the population meant that in the absence of such a basis, competition between practitioners was widespread. The effect, Larson (1977: 20) argues, was that we cannot speak of a single market for medicine but several markets, with different medical commodities being produced by different schools of healing such as allopathy and homeopathy. The controversies were bitter indeed, a state of affairs which lead a British observer to comment in the *Lancet* of 1860 on 'the very disunited state of the profession as evidenced form a mass of papers and reports in the Melbourne press . . . indeed, Melbourne and its hospital have certainly become famous in the annals of social-medical warfare'. There was even a case reported of a duel being fought between two doctors at Bendigo in 1861 following a disagreement over the treatment of hydatids. The *Medical Record* (Dec 1861: 135–136) reports:

> at first it was suggested that they fall back on the professional weapon of destruction — the scalpel; but as it was anticipated that they might be more fatally proficient with these than firearms, the/ latter mode was at last decided. Thursday evening, sundown, the plains of Bagshot were the time and place appointed, and at the hour and place were to be found the men, and the affair having got wind, a pretty large audience was gathered . . ., breathless was the interest as the distance, rather long by the way, some thirty or forty yards, was paced by the seconds. back to back stood the belligerents, until the word 'fire' raised the intensity of the feeling of the spectators to a pitch. At the word the fire flashed forth from the pistol of Dr . . .; but harmless was the effect. . . . his 'vis-a-vis' was seen pulling the trigger and countenance in every possible way and cursing the pistol that would not go off, and no wonder for as it afterwards appeared it had not been cocked. The seconds now interfered and the principals having declared their honour satisfied, the whole party returned homewards. In the course of the journey it oozed out, in some unexplainable manner, that the seconds, in loading the pistols, had omitted to put in those necessary ingredients — bullets, but whether from motives of mercy or from inexperience in affairs of honours, is not known.

Physical clashes also occurred between qualified and unqualified practitioners. Howden (1974: 191) reports cases of horsewhipping in the streets and court cases for assault on the goldfields involving practitioners.

Nor was the dividing line between qualified and unqualified practitioners clearly drawn. A visitor to Melbourne in 1853, William Kelly relates meeting a chemist in Emerald Hill (South Melbourne), and in conversation had his attention drawn to an advertisement in the window of the chemist's shop, selling 'the first class Dublin diploma of the late Dr . . .'. The chemist indicated that his business outlook was decent 'although somewhat dampened by the premature death of the M.D. on the hill, who "had slipped through in a bout of delerium tremens" '. On Kelly's disclaiming any medical knowledge, the chemist ventured:

> that in his opinion a tolerably smart man, of good address and general knowledge with a smattering of latin, would make a fair average colonial doctor. . . . Now and then . . . a bad lying-in case

occurs, but as the midwife is held responsible, the doctor need not be uneasy about the consequences.' As further encouragement 'he assured me that there were several doctors in and around Melbourne, in full practice, who never attended a lecture or smelt a subject, and more than one who compounded his own medicines, because he could not write a prescription'. (Kelly, 1859: 45)

That unqualified practitioners (dubbed 'quacks') flourished in early Victoria there is little doubt. Gandevia (1971: 56) suggests the reason for this being their cheapness, relative to qualified practitioners and thus preferred by 'the relatively impecunious working class'. 'Quacks' remained significant into the twentieth century and their role in minstering to the working class should not be underestimated or dismissed as a curious historical anachronism as most medical historians have tended to do. These unqualified practitioners found their way into popular culture, as this verse from the song 'Australian Humbugs' by the well-known and popular colonial songster Charles Thatcher would indicate.

The medical men without leave to kill,
Who doses you with black draught and blue pill,
And make you believe you're dreadfully ill,
    Are also Australian Humbugs.
Although ignorant of ailment or disease,
Each doctor tacitly agrees,
On every victim he can to seize,
And he never forgets to claim his fees.
The science of medicine is thus profaned,
By vilest quackery fortunes gained,
And the poor man's purse is frequently drained,
    By Australian Medical Humbugs.

(Thatcher, 1864: 163–164)

It's not clear that Thatcher's cynical wit applies only to unqualified practitioners either.

In this early period the division of labour was a very rudimentary one, consisting mainly of medical practitioners both qualified and unqualified. Conflict was a common within these two groups as it was between them. The only other health occupation present in significant numbers were pharmaceutical chemists. As Pensabene's (1980: 7–15) analysis shows, chemists of the time not only dispensed the prescriptions of doctors, but also provided some routine medical advice themselves, for those conditions the chemist considered not to require the attention of the doctor.

The transplantation of the English model of health care into Australia, meant that chemists were nominally subordinate to medicine, however the greater accessibility and relative cheapness of the chemist compared to the doctor, made the chemist a formidable competitor despite his nominal subordination. Only later with state intervention to legally restrict the supply of certain drugs to the provision of a doctors prescription did this substantially change. Chemists also contributed to another major feature of health care provision in this period, which also affected the demand for doctors' services, that being the tendency to self medication through patent medicines and remedies. Some chemists ran large and successful mail order businesses claiming to have patent medicines available which could cure almost every condition.

The major consequence of this competition, controversy and lack of effectiveness was a lack of public confidence in doctors which served as an impediment in their quest for political power and social status. On this question of status there is a disagreement within the literature. Medically qualified historians such as Gandevia (1971) have argued that social mobility for doctors was easily achieved in early Australia, and the doctor was able to assume an upper middle class position with greater ease than his counterparts elsewhere, especially in the United Kingdom. Without actually presenting much evidence to support his case Gandevia gives a number of reasons he sees as being important to this; including the experience of a ship voyage which promoted respect for the doctor (each migrant ship was required to carry one), and the effect of distances, the lack of a rigid class structure so that wealth rather than birth became the predominant means of judging 'social worth'. Others, such as McGrath (1975) have accepted Gandevia's argument without questioning.

Pensabene (1980) on the other hand argues that the professional power and status of the doctor was low in the nineteenth century and remained so until the impact of 'better' medical knowledge was felt in the twentieth century. As evidence Pensabene (1980: 33) cites the public questioning of the expertise of doctors in the press of the day. Some problems exist with the use of newspaper editorials as evidence of public opinion but both Gandevia and Pensabene fail to take adequate account of the segmentation of medicine of the day, particularly the distinction between the elite and the rank-and-file. This notion of segmentation is important to the analysis being made here. As Bucher and Strauss (1961) have argued, medicine has been and continues to be composed of a number of competing factions or segments and competition between these internal groups has affected its development. It is possible to show as Inglis (1958: 29) does, that doctors quickly became established as community leaders and had considerable involvement in the public affairs of early Victoria. Yet he is clearly referring (as is Gandevia) to the elite of the profession and his generalisation to the whole profession in arguing that doctors as a whole had high status (being the first professional men in the colony along with clergy), is unjustified in the light of the evidence provided by Pensabene. Likewise Pensabene is generalising from the rank-and-file segment to the occupation as a whole. The point seems to be that the elite, which became organised around the medical school (when it became established) and Collins Street, was the militant vanguard of the occupation, dragging the bulk of rank-and-file practitioners along with it, albeit at times reluctantly. Medicine thus reflected considerable status differences; the elite were able to draw upon traditional class mechanisms such as education to establish their positions, in a fashion similar to that demonstrated by Peterson in English society from where they had originated. The majority of qualified practitioners however had no such ideological resources available to them.

The professionalisation of medicine

The focus in this chapter is upon the production of medical dominance of the Victorian health system; that is the rise of medicine to a position of political and economic power. To examine this process, a distinction needs to be made for analytical purposes between two 'dynamics' of professionalisation, following Klegon (1978). The internal dynamic involves those actions related to attempts to regulate the occupation from within. Two features of this strategy exist; one involves the establishment of occupational associations to regulate the behaviour of individual practitioners, the other instituting a means of ensuring adequately trained entrants into the profession. The external dynamic by contrast involves the relationship of medicine to the wider political economy, in particular to the state through licensing laws and external regulatory mechanisms.

The external dynamic primarily involves consideration of the relationship between medicine and the state, through the introduction of licensing laws and their progressive refinement. The period 1840–1880 was marked in all western countries by the attempts of doctors to secure statutory registration (licensing) as a means of securing competitive advantage within the medical marketplace over other purveyors of medical commodities, such as homeopaths, patent medicine sellers and 'quacks'. As others (eg Larson, 1977: 20) have argued, the health arena was one in which the state was compelled to intervene early. This was because of the 'saliency' of the medical function in reflecting major features of the ideology of the post-feudal world (the value of human life and individualism). State sanctions thus represented an effort to standardise and regulate health practices and took place considerably before the rise of modern medicine (Larson, 1977: 20). Such an argument applies with some relevance in the Victorian context, though Larson tends to represent the relationship between the state and medicine as a fairly unproblematical one. In Victoria, the attempt by medicine to gain state patronage through licensing legislation went on for over a decade, and generally speaking was fairly minimal throughout the period under consideration.

The major impediment to securing legislation was an ideological one. 'Laissez-faire' individualism arose with the development of capitalism in the eighteenth and nineteenth centuries and stressed the desirability of state non-intervention in the economic world. Attempts to regulate the medical market were seen as inconsistent with this ideology and it was one of the most difficult factors for doctors to overcome in their attempts to secure market advantage over their competitors. As Davison (1978: 105) notes, politicians repeatedly affirmed their belief in free competition as the best regulator of professional practice, as well as other gainful activities. In the very early stages of settlement in Victoria, governmental regulation over the health area was minimal, as it was over other areas of social life. So long as he or she could attract patients, anyone could provide medical treatment (subject to criminal responsibility if harm or death resulted). Interestingly this is still the overall case in Victoria, although it is more hedged with other qualifications.

The earliest regulation related more to the need for the state to maintain legitimacy in the legal/justice area than to securing competitive advantages for doctors. The first Act was passed in 1838, after 50 years of settlement in Australia, when Victoria was still administered as part of New South Wales. This followed an English Act (1.Vic.-3.1838) in restricting the presentation of medical evidence at coroner's inquests to qualified practitioners. A few months later it was deemed necessary to define exactly who was 'qualified'. The NSW Medical Board was set up to administer the new act, which specified that in order to be deemed 'legally qualified', an applicant:

> must prove to the board he was a doctor or a bachelor of medicine in some university in the United Kingdon or Ireland, a member of the Apothecaries Society of London, a member of the college of physicians or surgeons in the United Kingdom or Ireland, or had served in the sea or land service. (2.Vic.22.1845)

Later, in 1844, an amendment was passed setting up a medical board for the district of Port Phillip (as Melbourne was then known), to save applicants the inconvenience of going all the way to Sydney to register their qualifications (8.Vic.8.1944). The board had no special powers and merely registered the qualifications of those who chose to present them and then published the list. Registration was not compulsory and a significant number who were qualified chose not to do so. Further amendments extended the provision of the Act to include practitioners trained in other specified places. All these acts however were concerned only with setting up a medical register for official purposes such as coroners' inquests. While this was important to the development of medicine's relationship with the state and as an institution of social control, the Acts were less important in influencing the evolution of the division of labour, since the rights of practice of other practitioners were not affected. Rather, the most important period deals with the events leading up to the first major registration Act— the Medical Practitioners Act of 1862 (24.Vic.158.1862).

The analysis of these events involves the internal dynamic of professionalisation; that is attempts to regulate the practice of medicine from within the profession itself. The earliest attempt at occupational organisation was in 1846 when the Port Phillip Medical Association was established to promote the interests of 'legally qualified' practitioners. The constitution of this body in fact predated that of both the British Medical Association and the American Medical Association. It lasted until 1851, when internal disagreements over ethical rules lead to its disbandment (MJA, 26.9.1936: 427). Several different organisations appeared after this. The Victorian Medical Association was set up in 1852, and determined to concentrate upon externally regulating practice by curbing the activities of unqualified practitioners, rather than deal with the internal issues such as ethical rules which had lead to the demise of the earlier association (MJA, 26.9.1836: 427). Soon after, in 1854, the Medico-Chirurgical Society was established, centered mainly around Melbourne hospital.

The transformation of the colony of Victoria which was brought about by the discovery of gold, had a considerable effect on the organisation of medical practice. For one thing it lead to the more rapid development of rural Victoria, especially around the goldfields, as large numbers of prospectors tried their hands. It also brought many practitioners, both qualified and unqualified into great competition with each other and lead to considerable pressure for reform as qualified practitioners strove to gain competitive advantage over their unqualified counterparts.

In 1853, Bowden (1974: 191) reports, a meeting of qualified practitioners was held on the goldfields at Castlemaine to discuss the activities of unqualified practitioners. This resulted in the formation of Castlemaine Medical Association. The association published lists of qualified practitioners in newspapers (eighteen on the first list published in August 1853), and on handbills which were distributed around the diggings. The name was changed in 1854 as the number of members grew, becoming the Mt Alexander Medical Association. In July 1854, the Bendigo District Medical Association was set up following the Mt Alexander example and a list containing eighteen names was published. Not all those eligible to join the new associations chose to, and this fact enable unqualified practitioners who were claiming to be qualified to continue doing so.

In 1855, the various associations amalgamated to form the Medical Society of Victoria (henceforth MSV), with the aim of jointly seeking restrictions on unqualified practice. Likewise a leading cause of the establishment of the *Australian Medical Journal*, begun in 1856, was the promotion of medical reform which included the suppression of quackery (Gandevia, 1952; McGrath, 1975). The MSV began to agitate for the compulsory registration of all qualified practitioners. In July 1856, a committee was established to draft a model bill to achieve this end. In October they presented such a bill to the Legislative Assembly for consideration. A major feature of their proposed bill was a ban on unqualified practice as well as the compulsory registration of all qualified practitioners (AMJ, 1856: 284–7). The attempt to secure legislation was not successful on this occasion and it was a further six years (1862) before legislation was passed, and then in a modified form to that proposed by the MSV.

In seeking registration, the doctors came up against a number of difficulties. The most important of these was the ideology of 'laissez-faire' individualism which ran counter to the notion of restricting economic activity in the health area to those who were 'duly qualified'. This ideology was invoked on many occasions. For example in a court case over the alleged mishandling of a childbirth at Bendigo in 1862, involving an unqualified practitioner by the name of Moody, the Crown claimed:

> it was incidental whether an accused person was properly qualified or whether he had been adequately educated for his profession. If he held himself capable of administering remedies, he was bound to use all care, attention and assiduity in his handling of a case, and if he did not do so, and exhibited culpable rashness, want of care or gross ignorance, he would be criminally responsible for the act if harm or death resulted. (*Bendigo Advertiser*, 1862, quoted by Bowden, 1974: 175)

The corollary of this was that it was the basic right of citizens to choose who to consult for their health and not a matter for state regulation.

The medical profession it should be noted, was by no means unified in its desire for registration and reform. Some doctors, responding to the ideology themselves, in fact openly argued against registration much to the annoyance of those pressing for it. One of the main opponents to the bill was Dr John Owens, a qualified practitioner and member of the Legislative Assembly. Owens believed that men who had been practising for some time had earned the right to continue their means of livelihood although their qualifications did not measure up to the standard required by the Medical Board (Bowden, 1974: 123).

The response of the doctors to the ideology of 'laissez-faire' individualism was to agree with the right of individuals to choose their own practitioner, but to argue in a somewhat patronising fashion that some were more capable of deciding than others. An early editorial in the *Australian Medical Journal* claimed:

> it is not that the wealthy and intelligent classes are prone to be duped by the nostrums of medical quackery—the evil is greater because the uninformed, the credulous, the poorer classes among whom afflication is far more serious and less easily alleviated, become the victims of a system of fraud, which perils life by its ignorance and recklessness and against which the public is offered neither protection nor redress. (AMJ, 1856: 51)

In so doing they also revealed their class orientation. Again in 1858, an editorial defended the right of people to choose who to consult, but added 'it is an imperative duty of the state to protect the labouring classes and especially the poor and uneducated classes from becoming the prey of ignorant and designing men' (AMJ, 1858: 203).

The internal dynamic or professionalisation was thus aimed at strengthening the case for state patronage. At this early stage however, the relationship with the state was still a fairly perfunctory one, and remained so throughout this period under consideration.

Another factor which appeared to obstruct the achievement of medical reform, was the seeming lack of public demand for the legislation. It was seen by many as a piece of self-interested legislation which few outside the profession itself wanted. In a pamphlet written in 1858, a doctor, APC Robertson, opposed reform because there was no public demand for it. His pamphlet and he himself were vilified subsequently in the *Australian Medical Journal* (1856: 276–280). Elsewhere in the same journal however the comment appears: 'medical questions are so little understood or appreciated by the public that every where there is great indisposition to medical legislation' (AMJ, 1856: 207).

Thirdly the internal disagreements mentioned above also contributed to the reluctance of the legislature. An editorial in the *Australian Medical Journal* in 1860, lamenting the lack of progress in achieving medical reform, commented, 'the legislature says it is ready to legislate as soon as the profession can agree on the kind and amount of legislation necessary. But the profession *will not* agree' (AMJ, 1860: 56–58; emphasis in original).

Fourthly, restrictions on unqualified practitioners would have deprived many outlying and isolated rural areas of any medical service at all as qualified practitioners were often reluctant to settle in these areas. This factor was probably less important in Victoria than it was in some other states such as Queensland, where medical registration was not compulsory until after 1880.

While concern that the best medical treatment was available to all was undoubtedly a major motive in pressing for registration, it is naive to think that this was the only or even the most important reason. Indeed statements such as the following should be viewed as part of the ideology of medicine of the era, in seeking to improve the rewards and status of the occupation.

... in thus claiming the protection of the legislature for the labourer and gold digger, let it not be supposed for a moment that we ask this protection from self interested motives. The medical profession in Australia wont nothing for themselves, they have nothing to ask for their own aggrandizement. (AMJ, 1858: 207)

Statements such as these, are contradicted by many others which help to show that the aim of registration was to secure an income and status advantage over other unqualified practitioners. Medical registration was needed, an editorial in the *Australian Medical Journal* (1856: 90) claimed, by the medical profession, 'to maintain and fortify its proper position in the social fabric'. Appeals to the state for market advantage were justified by class ideology. For example in the role it gave them in controlling access to charity:

there is no duty whatever more important in the affluent ranks of society, no obligation more sacred, than preserving the less rich, but no less independent classes below them, from imbibing those feelings of dependence on charitable assistance, for the enjoyment of advantage that, without such aid, are, with common prudence within reach of all. (AMJ, 1860: 27)

There was also the claim to special privileges in return for the role of medicine as an institution of social control in carrying out official duties.

The state that made a law demanding of us a protracted period of study before granting us a legal qualification to practise as a profession, should in simple justice, afford us by the same means a protection against those who infringe the law to the prejudice alike of the public and profession. (AMJ, 1856: 125)

All this should lead to a position of power and dominance within the health system, the editorial argued, 'our position as an important class within the community should enable us to dictate on all questions pertaining to our common interests' (AMJ, 1856: 91).

The passing of the English Act in 1858 undoubtedly hastened the passage of the Victorian legislation, as the colonial parliament looked to its English parent for precedents. The *Australian Medical Journal* saw the benefit of the English legislation too.

It will prove of eminent service to the Australian colonies by introducing amongst us a superior class of medical men, and, with higher scientific acquirements and greater professional skill, we feel assured that the medical profession in these colonies would enjoy, as a class, much more of the esteem and respect of the public than they have hitherto done. (AMJ, 1858: 209)

The English bill however contained provisions that had not been part of the bill that the Victorian profession had been pressing for. The English Act guaranteed (through the Privy Council) the rights to practise any theory of medicine or surgery and not just allopathy. No such provision was contemplated in the Victorian bill and its passage was frustrated particularly during 1858 and 1859 by Heales and Owens, the two main opponents of registration. Heales, appealing to the dominant ideology, wanted the protection of free trade in the medical area, which would protect the rights of homeopaths to practise. Owens did likewise, and in parliamentary debates despised the 'petty' animosities which characterised the profession in Australia arguing that 'if they were to pass a bill at all, it should only require that a man should show that he was a duly qualified practitioner, whatever his school might be' (quoted in AMJ, 1858: 241).

The English bill had also contained an 'infamous conduct' clause, which allowed for practitioners to be struck off the medical register for felonies or misdemeanours. Such a clause is important to the analysis being made here, in that it would allow internal regulation of medicine. In other words the supervisory body (later the Medical Board) made up of doctors could exercise control over the members of the profession through the threat of deregistration for 'infamous conduct', a phrase which could be interpreted in a variety of ways. Internal regulation I would argue, is the essential condition for autonomy (ie freedom from outside regulation or control, be it lay or governmental). Such internal regulation was not achieved finally in Victoria until 1933 and marks the end of the period in which the production of medical dominance is analysed. The *Australian Medical Journal* (1859: 48) however, was in favour of it from the time of the English Act; 'that the power was required was undeniable for instances have occurred where men did more dishonour it than the most atrocious or audacious' (AMJ, 1859: 48).

The legislation finally passed, in much amended form in 1862. It did not prevent unqualified practice but gave qualified practitioners considerable advantages. Only qualified practitioners could call themselves by medical titles, sue for non-payment of fees, hold official appointments and sign death certificates. A medical register was established, administered by the Medical Board and registration was required by qualified practitioners in order to take advantage of the benefits the act offered.

Importantly, the Act also contained as the English one had done, a 'grandfather' clause. This allowed those who had been trained by the apprenticeship system and who had been practising in Victoria since 1853, to register under the Act and enjoy its advantages, even though they did not hold any formal qualification in medicine, surgery or apothecary. The MSV opposed this clause but it was one of the amendments forced through by opponents of the bill in the legislature (especially Owens). However only nine practitioners subsequently registered under it (two per cent of the total).

The Act did not guarantee the right to practise any theory of medicine, as the English act had done, but neither did it restrict that right. The official duties of the profession were expanded to include the writing of the death certificates and holding government positions (such as coroner). In return for this state function, certain market advantages were bestowed upon it. The profession saw the main advantage of the act as restricting the right to use medical titles. An editorial in the *Australian Medical Journal* argued the Act had become 'the sole means of drawing the line between the educated possessor of an honorable title and the unscrupulous charlatan whose only qualifications are stupendous ignorance and boundless self assertion' (AMJ, 1862: 286).

However while the 1862 Act gave qualified practitioners certain market advantages, it was less successful in curbing the activities of unqualified practitioners, who soon developed means of getting around its provisions (such as calling themselves 'surgeon's assistants'). In 1864, and editorial in the *Australian Medical Journal* (1864: 55–56) lamented the ineffectiveness of the Act and called for more zeal on the part of the qualified to enforce it. Several successful prosecutions of unqualified practitioners were favourably commented upon, including one at Ballarat of an unqualified practitioner by the name of Butler in March 1864. In his defence, Butler claimed that he had been in practice twelve years, had never been charged with malpractice or manslaughter (as others had), had never been drunk (as some qualified practitioners had been), and would be ruined if prosecuted. His arguments were of no avail and he was fined the maximum penalty of £50 (AMJ, 1864: 82–83). There were calls from doctors for tightening the legislation but the consolidation of legislation in 1865 was mainly concerned with correcting an anomaly in the 1862 Act to allow armed forces medical personnel to continue in practice even though they may not be qualified (Medical Practitioners Statute, No 262, 1865).

Besides the successful external attempts to secure a competitive advantage over others in the medical marketplace through legislation, the other dynamic of professionalisation was aimed internally. There were two aspects to this. One was the development of occupational organisations to secure control over those already in practice. The other was the establishment of a training institution which would promote an adequately and uniformly trained supply of new entrants into medicine.

1862 was thus important in the development of the occupation of medicine in Victoria as the year in which the Melbourne Medical School took its first students. The university had been opened in 1855 and attempts to establish a medical school began almost immediately. The founder of the school was Anthony Colling Brownless, an ambitious surgeon of substantial private means. Freed from the necessity of making a daily living, he was able to devote his time to university matters and exerted a dominant influence over medical school affairs for the next 35 years until his death in 1897. The main feature of the medical course which Brownless proposed was its length—five years, when comparable English courses were only four. With the benefit of hindsight, modern historians (eg Blainey, 1958) have applauded this 'visionary' approach. In fact I believe the length of training must be seen more as part of the attempt to improve the status of doctors in early Australian society by professionalisation. As Freidson (1970b: 77–80) has commented, 'the content and length of training of an occupation including abstract knowledge or theory, is frequently a product of a deliberate action of those who are trying to show that their occupation is a profession and should therefore be given autonomy'.

The effect of the long training was of course class restrictive, as the local profession realised. The MSV sent a memo to the university council protesting that it would cause hardship to local medical students:

> it is the more necessary to consider these points because there is not here as at home in the U.K., a choice of schools wherein the less affluent may obtain on terms suited to their means, a complete medical and surgical education; students being compelled to either comply with the lengthened curricula here, or proceed to Great Britain, or foregoing the desire to enter the profession, leave the opportunities afforded here as a virtual monopoly to the wealthy. (Quoted in Russell, 1977: 214)

The extra time spent in training and paying fees before earning an income thus restricted entry to those whose families could afford to support them over a long period of time. Another effect which the MSV foresaw was that a considerable number of students went to Great Britain to do their medical degrees, especially to Edinburgh, where the length of training was shorter and the entrance requirements lower. Some of this group did a first year at Melbourne and then went overseas to complete their qualifications. The result was that the local medical school had little effect on the supply of doctors in its first decade. Up till 1880 only 47 graduates were produced and it was not until 1911 that the school provided the bulk of the new medical graduates when the English National Health Insurance Act ended the high inflow of British trained doctors.

The other aspect of the internal dynamic of professionalisation involved attempts at securing internal reform which aimed to unify medicine against competitors in the medical marketplace. This was a major strategy in the rise of the occupation to political and economic power, but again was relatively unsuccessful during this period. Segmentation was rife. The Victorian public was treated to several cases of court action involving one doctor against another, which lead the editor of the *Australian Medical Journal* (Aug. 1863: 90–91) to comment 'we believe these squabbles between medical men sink the profession in the eyes of the public'. The antagonisms cited in this editorial were carried on at inquests, in the newspapers and in the journals. In 1862, an opposing medical journal—the *Medical Record*—began publication, 'to support the dignity and interest of the profession against those members of it whose efforts for years have been to sink it' (*Medical Record*, 1875, quoted in Gandevia, 1952: 186).

Several sources of segmentation can be isolated. One developed as the local medical graduates began to appear on the scene and began to dilute the domination of the profession by British practitioners. Having all experienced the same training course of five years as against the variety of training courses of three or four years duration, the local graduates were a more unified and homogeneous group and their influence grew steadily. Some antagonism towards them from British trained practitioners was encountered as a result. One occasion was in 1876 when the Melbourne Hospital administration, dominated by practitioners with British training refused to recognise the Melbourne degree as a basis for appointment to the position of surgeon at the hospital. The controversy which ensued was eventually solved (in favour of the local graduates) by an amendment to the Act so that after 1879 all local graduates received both a Bachelor of Medicine (MB) and a Bachelor of Surgery (BS) (Russell, 1977: 53).

A more important source of segmentation however was that between the hospital oriented academic elites and the rank-and-file of general practitioners. The *Australian Medical Journal* for example was criticised as the organ of a small and influential elite oriented around the university, the Melbourne hospital and the Collins Street practitioners. Pensabene (1980: 81) has calculated that 53 per cent of the presidents of the MSV between 1852 and 1906 practised in Collins Street and a further 24 per cent in the city of Melbourne. The *Medical Record* saw its role as representing the rest of the profession and claimed 'the sympathy of members of the Medical Society for the suffering public was as genuine as that which crows would express were they able to speak for sick lambs' (quoted in Gandevia, 1952: 186).

The *Medical Record* did not last long, but other journals such as the *Australian Medical Gazette* began publication later. In a libel suit against the publishers of the *Australian Medical Journal* a lawyer was moved to comment 'there were two sections of medical men in the colony who were continually abusing each other and they could not meet in consultation over a toothache without quarrelling' (quoted in McGrath, 1975: 139). An example of the hostility is the decision of the coroner (a doctor—Richard Youl) to assign all post-mortems to two members of the hospital and medical school elite; Halford and Neild. This act was viewed with great hostility by the doctors as depriving them of a potential source of income.

Hostility was also expressed over the attempts, mainly by the leadership of the MSV, to reduce competition between doctors. There were attempts early in the period to institute ethical rules as we have seen. Most of these dealt with seeking to internally regulate competition. This was a difficult task however and one which lead to the demise of the early medical association. The ethical rule most sought after was a ban on advertising which would have effectively prevented price cutting. Without the opportunity to advertise cheap prices the competition would not be as great. Advertising was defined as 'unprofessional conduct' (ie more suited to a trade than a profession). In 1860 Dr McKenna advertised a reduced scale of charges in the press and also placed cards under doors in an attempt to increase his practice. The controversy which followed lead to his resignation from the MSV (McGrath, 1975: 137). A ban on advertising however most favoured the elite of the profession at the expense of the bulk of the practitioners. With 'honorary' hospital posts the elite were quite visible anyway and thus did not need to advertise. The practitioner most affected was the general practitioner attempting to start up in practice or to increase his workload. A ban thus severely restricted his ability to do so, especially when as Pensabene (1980) has argued, concern with overcrowding was being expressed frequently in the medical press.

The different interests of these rival sections eventually lead to the establishment of a rival professional association. Dr James Henry had resigned from the MSV over a disagreement in 1878 and went to England. On his return he carried with him authorisation papers to set up the Victorian Branch of the British Medical Association, which he did in 1879. The MSV accepted its rival (having little choice) arguing the new association could concentrate on medical politics and ethical discipline, leaving the MSV to concentrate on scientific matters. However despite considerable overlap of membership, disharmony between the two organisations soon emerged and persisted until they were finally united in 1911.

The other major source of segmentation which existed concerned the state of medical knowledge at the time. A division of opinion existed over the source of infectious diseases (or zymotic diseases as they were then known). This was particularly relevant as Melbourne suffered from epidemics of various infectious diseases including typhoid, diptheria (in children), erysipelas (also known as 'hospitalism'). Without a secure body of medical theory a diversity of beliefs about the cause of disease was possible. In broad terms, and at the risk of oversimplifying the controversies there were two major theories. A lot of practitioners (Pensabene, 1980: 22, argues a majority) believed in the spontaneous origin of infectious diseases. These practitioners, known as miasmists, believed that infectious disease was spontaneously generated from a miasma of dead and decaying matter and condemned the poor state of Melbourne's sanitation and drainage (the major public health issue in the latter part of the nineteenth century), as the principal source of infectious diseases. Contagionists on the other hand were early adherents of the germ theory, believing that germs and bacteria were the cause of infectious diseases. These theories of course were not peculiar to Victoria but were representative of a much wider debate going on throughout the Western medical world.

The confusion over the origin of disease resulted in a variety of treatments as well, with miasmists advocating public health measures such as the effective sanitation and water treatment, and exposure to fresh air for those who had already contracted the disease. Contagionists on the other hand prescribed large and often chaotic mixtures of drugs. The debate raged for more than a decade. The *Australasian Medical Gazette* (April, 1893) commented 'every man seems to have his theory—hardly any two persons are agreed regarding the conditions favouring (disease) production'.

Of course this disagreement did not improve the public image of the profession as this *Age* editorial (27.1.1875: 2) indicates: 'it would be too much to expect that doctors should agree on any given subject arising out of their science and the board of health cannot make up its mind to say whether the germ theory of the causation of the disease is correct or whether it is propagated by the presence of dirt alone'. Infectious diseases were not the only area of disagreement or hazardous treatment. Surgery, the other major area where new technology was to have a major impact, was also unreliable and dangerous. Amputations were the most common operation and a major ordeal in pre-anaesthesia times when reliance was made on alcohol or opium to deaden the pain. Inglis (1958) reports that screams and cries from within the Melbourne hospital could be heard by anyone passing by on the street. The danger of post-operative infection was also very great.

A third theory of disease and treatment came from homeopaths. Some early homeopaths had medical training but for the most part homeopathy developed in competition with both miasmatic and contagionist theories practised by members of the various medical occupational associations. The 'sect' of homeopathy from the 1850s constituted the main threat to the dominance of 'orthodox medicine' or allopathy though other modalities existed of what we would call today alternative healing, including herbalism and electromagnetism.

John B Hickson and Thienette de Berigny were the two earliest practitioners of homeopathy in Victoria. Hickson began practice in 1850 and de Berigny arrived in Melbourne in the mid 1850s. The theory of homeopathy had been developed by a German doctor, Samuel Hahnemann, who in 1796 had proclaimed his theory that 'like cures like'; that disease could be cured by administration of a drug whose artificially induced range of symptoms resembled the symptom complex of the disease. The disease would be driven out by a similar artificially induced disease (Kaufman, 1971). The method of treatment which this theory advocated contrasted greatly with and developed as a revulsion to, allopathy. Whereas allopathy preached the theory of opposites and at the time used large drug doses, homeopathy, in response to what it saw as this overtreatment used highly attenuated doses of drugs, much diluted and of very low potency. Homeopaths were often (derisively) referred to as 'globulists' by allopaths as a result.

In Victoria homeopathy gained a wide following and became a serious competitor to allopathic or orthodox medicine well into the twentieth century. It was hailed as the new 'scientific' art of healing (Templeton, 1969) and received many laudatory comments in the daily newspapers of the time. The *Age* for instance commented 'homeopathy is now patronised by nearly all the educated classes of Europe and America—emperors, kings, queens, ambassadors, statesmen, archbishops, philosophers, journalists etcetera' (quoted by Templeton, 1969: 9). Amongst its supporters in Melbourne were the Dean of Melbourne, the Very Reverend Hussey Burg Macartney, the Lord Bishop of Melbourne, the Right Reverend Charles Perry and the Chief Justice of Victoria, William Forster Stawell (Inglis, 1958: 44). The practice of homeopathy was not confined to Melbourne either, a letter to the *Australian Medical Journal* in 1865, written by a country practitioner, claimed of homeopathy, 'it injures our pockets as well as our characters' (AMJ, 1865: 56).

Homeopaths thus constituted the main competition for orthodox medicine in its rise to political and economic power and its control was a major step in the achievement of medical dominance. Homeopathy was attacked as the 'new medical heresy' (despite the internal segmentation of medicine itself) and homeopaths excluded from membership of the MSV even when they had initial medical training. The *Australian Medical Journal* in 1864 called it 'the emanation of a diseased mind, the product of an overwrought imagination and the foolish craze of an amiable madman' (AMJ, 1864: 245).

Opposition was expressed to any form of professional association, saying that 'between the globulistic quackery and rational medicine there can be no alliance (AMJ, 1873: 224). People who supported homeopathy were described as 'weak-minded' (AMJ, 1874: 23). Homeopathy constituted a particular threat furthermore because of its fashionable status, considerable community support and the fact that many homeopathic practitioners had been 'converted' from allopathy.

Through the 1870s and 1880s the controversy between homeopathy and allopathy raged in the newspapers and journals. The homeopaths saw themselves as pioneers, as founders of a new paradigm of medical knowledge, and thus put opposition from orthodox medicine down to professional jealousy and prejudice. Furthermore such opposition served only to strengthen their missionary zeal. Templeton (1969: 47) suggests that the scorn heaped upon homeopathy by the medical profession during the 1870s including the expulsion of those medically qualified from the MSV, little affected its popularity and probably increased it. Homeopaths attempted unsuccessfully to have a ward of Melbourne hospital converted to being run on homeopathic treatment lines despite considerable public support from hospital subscribers. Having failed, they then established their own homeopathic hospital in 1869 and during the 1880s scored a considerable victory in establishing a fully fledged homeopathic hospital (now Prince Henry's), which continued treatment along homeopathic lines until the 1930s. Not until 1906 when legislation was passed which had the effect of restricting the number of new homeopathic practitioners that could be registered in Victoria to one per year, was dominance over homeopathy effectively gained by orthodox medicine.

Despite the intense competition between homeopaths and allopaths however, I believe most historical accounts have tended to over-emphasise the differences between the two sects of medicine. Templeton (1969: 9) for example suggests that the extent to which Victorian homeopaths slavishly followed the teachings of the founder was open to question. The attachment of most to homeopathy she argues, was based more on pragmatism than theory as it appealed to those who liked interfering with nature as little as possible, and who despaired of the inadequacies of orthodox medicine at the time before the establishment of the germ theory of disease.

The debate between the sects and indeed between miasmism and contagionism was largely over the effects of various treatments rather than the theoretical incompatibility between them. Rather than homeopathy and allopathy being different paradigms of medical knowledge, I would argue, following the discussion in the previous chapter, they should both be seen as part of the same Individualist mode of medical production. The differences between them were primarily marketing differences; allopathy prescribed large doses of drugs and used bleeding as a form of treatment, homeopathy did not bleed and prescribed minimal drugs.

The medical profession in 1880

By 1880 then, medicine had a high-status, reasonably politically effective vanguard-elite who utilised their class positions and contacts in the political sphere to further the cause of the occupation as a whole (the external dynamic) while attempting to regulate and reform it from within (the internal dynamic). The efforts to professionalise received partial sanction from the state as part of an attempt to regulate and standardise the medical commodity. The relationship between medicine and the state however was quite a perfunctory one and was probably related more to a class affinity with the elite of the occupation than demonstrable claims of effectiveness. By 1880 however medicine was established in a strategic, if not entirely dominant position vis-a-vis homeopathy. In a simple division of health labour, medicine held a considerable competitive advantage over other health practitioners. The hierarchy of health workers was thus established prior to the introduction of new medical technology and medicine was in a strategic position to exploit the developments in medical knowledge which followed.

Entry to medicine was also by this time becoming more class restrictive as Davison (1978: 90–97) has argued. It required substantial family backing involving the purchase of both a private school and university education. Once qualified there were further costs which heightened this class restrictiveness, such as the cost of setting up in practice. As a result, three quarters of native born doctors who commenced practice during the 1880s were sons of professional men (Davison, 1978:96). Such a finding is corroborated by Pensabene's (1980: 70) analysis of obituary notices in the *Medical Journal of Australia*.

4 Technical and political processes in the rise of scientific medicine

This chapter examines the second part of the production of medical dominance. It examines the effects of the introduction of new medical knowledge and technology on medicine, its position within the health arena and with regard to the state. In conventional medico-historical terms the process to be analysed is the rise of 'scientific medicine'. In this study that process is conceptualised as a discontinuity in paradigms associated with the mode of production of medical commodities. Such a discontinuity can be temporally located as originating in the middle decades of the nineteenth century although conceptually the process was carried out over the whole period under consideration. The discontinuity in the modes of medical production was associated with the development of a new technology of medical work, based upon developments in the understanding of disease and the means for treating those disease. In Kuhn's (1970) terms a 'scientific revolution' occurred, in which there was a paradigm shift in the understanding and treatment of disease. The new paradigm which was instituted has come to be called the germ theory—the tracing of the causes of diseases to specific etiological agents (germs) which can be identified and treated or cured through either biological means (vaccines) or chemical means (drugs). Germ theory has come to provide the theoretical underpinning for what is referred to as 'scientific medicine'.

In this chapter I shall argue, contrary to technological determinist explanations that the development of this new technology of medical work was a necessary but not sufficient explanation for the achievement of medical dominance. Also crucial to medicine's success were factors external to the medical system itself, in particular those resulting from the nature of the social formation in Victoria of the time, and the stratified set of class relationships which emerged from that social formation. In other words primacy cannot be accorded to the internal dynamic of professionalisation. Instead the success of the internal dynamic could only be achieved within the political and economic context associated with the external dynamic. The professionalisation of medicine was associated with changes in the capitalist mode of production from laissez-faire to monopoly forms (see

Larson, 1977: 209). In the medical arena this transformation was reflected in the transformation in the mode of medical production. In turn, the transformation of the mode of medical production affected the changes in the mode of production of the society as a whole. The relationship in other words is a dialectical one, though one in which the economic changes in the society have overall primacy.

Although some historians such as Russell (1977: 16) have argued that medicine was becoming more scientific from much earlier than 1880, that date is chosen, for example by Pensabene (1980), as representing a qualitative break from the past. After 1880 there were fairly rapid developments in the understanding of disease and these developments were adopted and utilised by allopaths in their rise to political and economic power. As Rosenberg (1971: 22–35) has argued for the United States, and would appear to apply equally in the Australian context, doctors hitched their fortunes to the rising star of science. Appeals to the rationality of science as the basis of authority, Larsen (1977: 137) argues, became an important new ideology legitimating the social order.

The development of new medical technology

A scientific revolution, Kuhn (1970) argues, is always a highly political process. Dissatisfaction with the old paradigm grows over a period of time as more and more problems emerge which cannot be explained using the old paradigm. The existence of these anomalies eventually leads to a 'scientific revolution' which replaces the old paradigm with a new one. In the case of medicine, what were later hailed as major inventions were often around for long periods as such anomalies before they were totally accepted. For example the two discoveries which are regarded as crucial to the development of scientific medicine by many writers had both occurred earlier but were not generally accepted until much later. These were Pasteur's demonstration of the existence of germs in 1862 and Lister's application of that principle to surgical techniques in 1867.

New developments, discoveries, inventions in the medical field almost all took place out of Australia and mainly in Europe, though there was usually a time lag of only a few months between the publication of a new discovery and trials being conducted in Australia, or more particularly, in Victoria. Yet trials, even successful ones, did not mean the immediate acceptance of the new technique or treatment; in fact medical history books are full of stories about discoveries, 'ahead of their time', the discoverers of which were scorned at the time of their breakthrough, only to be recognised at a later date.

Surgery was the first major area where new developments were felt.

The first surgical use of ether as an anaesthetic was made in August 1847 by David Thomas at Melbourne hospital, only ten months after it had been first used by Morton in the United States (Potter, 1938: 940–949), though as Davidson (1968: 62) points out, its usefulness had been known as early as 1815. Chloroform temporarily replaced ether after being first used in 1848 (Potter, 1938: 940–949), though its negative side effects led to a return to ether later. The major development however was Lister's work, published in 1867. Lister had applied Pasteur's theory of the germ creation of disease to the surgery area and advocated antiseptic and aseptic surgery as a means of overcoming the post-operative infection which resulted in many deaths. Antiseptic surgery was first used in Victoria by William Gillies in December 1867 (Graham, 1952: 277). One might have expected wide adherence to fairly quickly follow, but there was considerable disagreement with Lister's techniques, partially because the antiseptic he advocated (carbolic acid) was a fairly inefficient one, and in fact antiseptic surgery was little used till the 1880s and not fully applied until the late 1880s (Lee, 1944: 653), as the epidemics of erysipelas in 1882 and pyaemia in 1886 would indicate. There is also illustration of the Kuhnian argument that complete adherence to the new paradigm is not gained until the old practitioners have died out. Sir Thomas Fitzgerald, the famous Melbourne hospital surgeon, Inglis (1958: 56–62) indicates, never accepted Lister's methods, or applied them only grudgingly and partially, practising with a high degree of success (apparently because of considerable dexterity and skill) until his death in 1908 (see also Russell, 1977: 107). Thus 40 years elapsed between the first surgical case in which antiseptic techniques were followed, until the last one in which they were not. As antiseptic techniques were gradually introduced hospitalism gradually ceased to be of major concern. Pensabene (1980: 37) has calculated that the number of deaths due to hospitalism dropped from twenty in 1875 (from 312 cases) to only one in 1895 (from 81 cases). Advances were also made in the instruments available in surgery. The Spencer Wells clamp for instance, introduced in 1872, made control of haemorrhage much easier (Lloyd, 1968: 36). With surgery safer and (slightly) less of an ordeal, other procedures could be attempted, especially in the area of abdominal surgery. The first appendectomy was carried out in 1887, the first in Victoria in 1893 (Lee, 1944: 657). Previously death had been almost inevitable from peritonitis.

The other major development was in the understanding of the source of disease, particularly infectious disease. Pasteur provided the basis for the development of the germ theory in 1862, challenging the spontaneous origin theory by demonstrating the role of micro-organisms. 'Proof' of the role of germs was provided by Koch in 1876 with his growing of the anthrax bacilli in an artificial medium (Crellin,

1968: 57–76). Once the methodology for isolating the micro-organisms that produced disease had been developed, the bacilli that caused infectious diseases were soon discovered so that by 1886, Castiglioni (1958: 817–818) demonstrates, the bacilli many diseases had been isolated. These included pneumonia, meningitis, gonorrhoea, tuberculosis, typhoid and diphtheria. However these discoveries did not immediately flow through into medical practice; knowing what caused a disease was much different from knowing how to treat it. Also many members of the British and Victorian profession were unconvinced by the discoveries and still clung to the theory of spontaneous creation of disease. Thus the controversy and public disputes continued which had characterised the medical scene in Victoria during the nineteenth century. Although Thomson, the main supporter of the germ theory, could claim in 1896 that 'the germ theory of the origin of zymotic disease is now accepted by even the most skeptical' (*The Age*, 2.3.1896: 4), the actual practical implications of such theoretical adherence had yet to affect the health of the people. Pensabene (1980: 43) has calculated that the death rate from contagious diseases (tuberculosis, diphtheria and typhoid) remained high throughout the late nineteenth century and in fact increased from 13.49 deaths per thousand in 1871 to 17.76 deaths per thousand in 1889.

Explaining this apparent paradox between improving knowledge about disease on the one hand, and general lack of effectiveness for the population as a whole on the other, is facilitated by an understanding of the segmentation of medicine, in particular between the elite and the rank-and-file. While there were some exceptions (such as Fitzgerald), the elite, centred around Collins Street, Melbourne hospital and the medical school, appear to have accepted readily the new developments and technology resulting from these, and began socialising new entrants into the paradigm at the medical school from the 1880s. However the extent to which these new developments filtered through to the rank-and-file practitioners who numerically constituted the bulk of the occupation, is less certain.

To understand this phenomenon further, I believe one of the lasting insights provided by Eliot Freidson, detailed previously, is useful. In the training which doctors receive, Freidson (1970b: 165–166) argues, two types of knowledge are stressed. One is book knowledge or theoretical knowledge; the other being knowledge gained from experience, or clinical knowledge. In Freidson's account of training, textbook knowledge was constantly treated as inferior to knowledge from experience (even in the 1960s), and knowledge from experience was considered a valid counter-argument to 'scientific' knowledge. Thus the actual practice of medicine becomes a result of the application of these two types of knowledge, with clinical knowledge taking priority over book knowledge (developing what Freidson terms the 'clinical mind').

Applying this insight historically, one might argue that the Individualist mode in which the practitioners of the day had been trained would, in the virtual absence of effective or agreed upon theoretical knowledge, have relied even more strongly on clinical knowledge. With new developments in textbook or theoretical knowledge, the bulk of practitioners preferred to continue practising on the basis of their accumulated experience, especially when better understanding of disease had not been translated into more effective treatment (see Rothstein, 1972: 256–266). This incidentally is not to imply any negative value connotation to this action; indeed one might argue that a healthy degree of skepticism towards developments in medical practice is neither reactionary nor irrational, but a reasonable position. This would be particularly the case where new developments were introduced in a fairly crude form (eg ether) before refinement took place.

Furthermore the apparent paradox in the resistance to scientific medicine can be explained in terms of there being less commensurability between allopathy and scientific medicine than is usually assumed. Although most allopaths came to practise scientific medicine, allopathy did not just evolve into scientific medicine. Certainly it used the term 'scientific' for the legitimacy attached to that term, but there is a qualitative difference between allopathy (or what I have called the Individualist mode) and scientific medicine (the Corporatist mode), as detailed in a previous chapter. The resistance to scientific medicine was understandable at this early stage in which it appeared quite different from that with which many practitioners were familiar.

Clearly what was necessary was a translation of a better understanding of the *theory* of disease into practical terms in the form of *treatment*. This led during the 1880s to the search for antitoxins as a means of preventing and treating infectious disease. The first antitoxin was developed in 1890 by Behring for diphtheria (Castiglioni, 1958: 824), and trials were first carried out in Victoria in the Melbourne suburb of Hawthorn in 1897 (Cresswell, 1897: 1775–1798). There was great interest in Victoria also in 1890 when Koch announced he had isolated the antitoxin for tuberculosis. *The Argus* (3.11.1890: 6) hailed it as 'the greatest triumph that medical science has ever achieved' and a member of the local medical elite, Springthorpe, travelled to Europe to investigate it. However, tuberculin (as the antitoxin was called) was found not to be as successful as had been hoped and a cure for tuberculosis was in fact still many years away (Maddox, 1937: 801).

Developments in the technology of medical work also occurred in the area of diagnosis. In 1896 Roentgen first published his findings on the use of X-rays to detect foreign bodies and internal injuries, and in the treatment of fractures. Within a few months trials were carried out at the University of Melbourne and X-rays gradually came into usage (Eddy, 1946: 143). Further important developments occurred during the early twentieth century, the most important of which appears to have been the foundation of chemotherapy with the work of Ehrlich in isolating the first synthetic arsenical compound 'salvarson'. This was found to be useful in the treatment of syphilis. In 1911 radium was used to treat cancer for the first time (Bray, 1939: 849). Over the period in question then new developments were gradually introduced into medical practice and the establishment of the new paradigm began.

Effectiveness and impact

While the developments outlined above constituted major advances in the technology of medical work, the question of their effectiveness in reducing mortality in the population as a whole is open to question. Certainly in some areas such as surgical techniques, considerable advantages were very obvious, but the benefit is less obvious with regard to the major causes of mortality of the age. As we have seen, at least until the end of the nineteenth century mortality rates for major infectious diseases such as measles, diphtheria, typhoid and tuberculosis remained high, so that the death rate as a whole actually rose. Infant mortality rates also rose slightly in the same period, from 121.5 to 126.8 deaths per thousand (Victorian Yearbooks).

In other words while the germ theory gradually became firmly established in the sense of gaining the widespread support of doctors, it was unable to provide specific treatment especially for infectious diseases, at least prior to 1890. From the turn of the century however mortality, especially from infectious diseases, did begin to decline substantially. The death rate as a whole fell from 16.09 deaths per thousand in 1890 to 8.93 deaths by 1930. The reduction in mortality in some areas was even more striking; for instance among young children as Gandevia (1978: 729) has shown. Rates of other infectious diseases also declined. Apparently 'scientific medicine', utilising the germ theory, had become effective. Yet this effectiveness I believe to be highly questionable and I propose to consider this issue in some detail.

In an important article entitled 'On the Limitations of Modern Medicine' (1973), Powles argues, in the English context, that although scientific medicine, in particular chemotherapy, has been effective in some specific areas such as pain relief, it has generally been much less effective than is claimed. In particular, it has been less important in contributing to declining mortality than public health factors such as improvements in diet, living conditions etc. Examining a range of infectious diseases, he shows that the major decline in the mortality rates from these various infectious diseases occurred prior to the introduction of specific chemotherapeutic agents. Publication of this seminal work led to further work in other Western countries such as the USA (McKinlay and McKinlay, 1977), but similar issues have not been closely examined in the Australian context. However, some evidence has become available which allows a secondary analysis to be undertaken, and similar conclusions to those made by Powles can be tentatively made pending a more thorough investigation. Several areas can be examined.

First, Sinclair (1975) has examined death rates from typhoid in Melbourne from 1870 to 1914. He concludes that the decline in typhoid death rates during that period were largely unrelated to advances in scientific medicine. Instead they were related more to social and environmental factors, in particular improved water supplies, drainage and sanitation. Secondly, in his analysis of the decline of age specific mortality rates, Gandevia (1978) concludes that 80 per cent of the decline was due to the reduced incidence of the disease itself rather than specific therapeutic developments, which he argues 'appear to have played no major role in the reduction of any of the infectious diseases' (Gandevia, 1978: 132). He goes on to argue that this did not mean therapeutic techniques such as diptheria antitoxin were ineffective, 'but for the most part mortality had fallen to such low levels, or was already falling so markedly that no deflection of a graphic trend is detectable' (Gandevia, 1978: 132).

Much earlier research by Armstrong (1939) had concluded that the lowered mortality rate was largely the result of improvements in economic conditions which had the effect of raising the standard of living. He cites the change from bottle to breast feeding as contributing also. With regard to diphtheria, measles and consumption, Cumpston (1927) has demonstrated that the changing incidence of these diseases can be explained more by changes in the age composition of the population than by specific medical treatments.

Now this is not necessarily to imply that doctors themselves were uninvolved in improvements in the nation's health, in particular the declining death rate. Indeed members of the medical profession were deeply involved in public health measures such as the sanitary reform movement and the Australian Health Society founded in 1875. But these movements which appear to have been more responsible for better health, along with better diet etc, relied for the most part not on the germ theory but on the 'unscientific' miasmatic theory (VPP, 2, 1890: 17-76).

The consequences of miasmists' concern with sanitation and public health measures appear to have been a reduction in mortality, however 'wrong' they may have been about the causes of disease. The improvement in health, in other words, appears to have been more of an unintended consequence of theories of disease causation such as miasmatic ones than as a result of the germ theory. Nonetheless, medicine was able to claim the improvements in health as being the result of the new technology of medical work and, as Pensabene (1980: 49) argues, this 'favourable coincidence that the revolution in medicine and surgery was paralleled by an equally revolutionary decline in mortality' facilitated the rise in the 'professional status' of medicine. The important point to be made here is that 'scientific medicine' (which was based upon the germ theory) became established (in the sense of acquiring dominance) in the absence of clear evidence of its effectiveness. The claim to effectiveness, drawing on the supposed past record of control over infectious diseases, has become part of the ideology of medicine, only recently dented by the work of Powles and others.

Finally in this section on developments in medical knowledge, it is important to note that although 'scientific medicine' has often been assumed to have been established by the second decade of the twentieth century, by modern standards the level of understanding and treatment of disease was very rudimentary. A retired Melbourne doctor, reminiscing about the 1920s, recalled:

> In those days there were no antibiotics and except for the anti-syphilitic arsenicals, no other specific chemotherapeutic agents against any of the microbic diseases, and our wards always contained cases, sometimes many cases of severe pneumonia, osteomyelitis, erysipelas, infected wounds, bacterial endocarditis and typhoid fever. Lacking specific remedies for any of these, our treatment was mainly good nursing while the disease ran its course . . . a considerable proportion of patients died . . . Tuberculosis was rife. (Willis R & M: *LTL Ms* 9877: 110–111)

Surgery, he says, was also very different from the present day:

> For all major operations we gave liquid ether, chloroform or mixtures of these on an open mask held over the patient's face. Induction was nearly always distressing for both patient and anaesthetist, and maintenance for a long operation demanded great experience and unrelaxed vigilance. Post operative vomiting was very common and often prolonged, not only depriving the patient of nourishment and rest but also causing severe pain from abdominal incisions. (Willis R & M: *LTL Ms* 9877: 112–113)

It was L J Henderson of Harvard University who claimed that 1912 was 'the first year in human history in which the random patient with a random disease consulting a random physician had a better than

50/50 chance of benefitting from the encounter' (quoted in Carter, 1958: 27).

The development of state patronage

Having examined the transformation in the technology of medical work in the previous section, I now propose to consider the development of the relationship between medicine and the state, in particular events leading to the position of dominance achieved by practitioners of scientific medicine with the passing of legislation in 1908. Medical dominance, it will be argued, was established by legislation in 1908 but not consolidated until further legislation in 1933. The crucial feature of this dominance is self government, internal to the occupation itself through an institution comprised entirely of medical practitioners. This body is the Medical Board of Victoria (henceforth MBV). Such internal self government establishes autonomy, the essential condition for professionalism as a form of control over work.

Although in this chapter I have analysed in some detail the developments in medical knowledge and technology, the process of state recognition is related to other factors than just those technical developments. As a previous chapter argued, social and political factors are important in the development of knowledge and the issue becomes one of the legitimacy of that knowledge. This is not to deny the importance of the 'discoveries', but to argue that medicine was able to use these, as well as the ideological arguments which came to be based upon them, to seek legitimation with the state. In other words, also important in the rise of 'scientific medicine' were social and political processes, such as the claim to effectiveness in reducing mortality from infectious diseases. This attempted to attribute such changes to the achievements of medical science in order to bolster the claim to state patronage.

This argument provides the framework for the analysis of the social and political processes in the production of medical dominance which follows. It should be noted however that such an argument is at variance with that made by Pensabene (1980), whose account tends to emphasise the role of new medical knowledge and technology. As a result, in the analysis which follows I will be both using and reconstructing his argument to show how the rise of medicine must be related more to social and political developments than to technical ones.

The phenomenon of medical dominance was produced in two stages; the first culminating in 1908, the second in 1933. Medical legislation passed prior to 1880 gave the medical profession certain market advantages, but it did not prevent from practising, other practitioners who were unqualified in the terms of the Act. In fact there is plenty of evidence to suggest that the passage of the various medical Acts of 1862 and its modification in 1865 did little to diminish the practise by 'unqualified' practitioners. Of this group homeopaths constituted the major threat to medicine and as we have seen in the previous chapter the controversy between allopaths and homeopaths which got underway in the 1860s continued into this period, a notable victory for the homeopaths in the 1880s being the opening of their own hospital.

During the 1880s and 1890s the doctors' dissatisfaction with the acts grew as 'unqualified practitioners' continued to practice and thrive. The penal provisions of the earlier acts were either not enforced, or when enforced resulted in minimal fines, much to the chagrin of the *AMJ* (15.3.1894: 151–152). Internal self regulation was first advocated by doctors in 1871, when the MSV wanted the right to be able to erase names of qualified practitioners for 'disreputable conduct', as well as to exclude those with questionable titles (AMJ, March 1871: 85). However medicine was unsuccessful in achieving any further legislative advantage until 1908.

Moreover in 1878 an attempt was made by supporters of 'unqualified' practitioners to deregulate the practice of medicine and erode even the partial market advantage which medicine enjoyed at the time. A private member's bill, the Medical Practitioners' Statute Amendment Bill, was unsuccessfully introduced which allowed for registration in any case of regular medical training followed by medical practice during the previous fifteen years in Victoria. A number of practitioners, particularly Chinese herbalists, would have been eligible for registration on this basis. There was considerable support for the bill in the legislature with its proponents pointing to the low technical skills of qualified practitioners. The MBV was adamently opposed to this dilution of the regulation of medicine, but the bill reached a second reading before being defeated (VPD, 16.10.1878: 1383).

Unsuccessful attempts were made by the MSV to have unqualified practice of medicine banned, most notably in 1892. These were vocally opposed by supporters of unqualified practitioners with 'laissez-faire' ideology invoked as the main objection (VPD, 2.8.1892: 742) and a petition of four to five thousand signatures presented to support these arguments.

During the latter part of the nineteenth century then, doctors were particularly unsuccessful in achieving their aim of dominance within the medical system. Patronage of unqualified practitioners remained high through this period encouraged by a number of factors. The class basis of medical care was one of these. A doctor's consultation fee (ten shillings and sixpence) constituted up to one third of the weekly wage of a manufacturing worker in the late nineteenth century (Pensabene, 1980: 154). The private services of doctors were thus only available to a very restricted sector of the public. Severe restriction of unqualified practice would have robbed a substantial proportion of the population of medical care in particular the large number of unemployed and poor created by the depression of the 1890s which had followed the boom period of the 1880s. Also in rural areas qualified practitioners were sometimes unavailable at all.

Several courses of action were available to those who could not afford the fees charged by qualified practitioners. Chemists have historically always been the practitioners of first contact for many conditions, as the 'poor man's doctor'. To get medical treatment one could join a friendly society or 'lodge', an institution transplanted into Victoria from England which provided cheap if rather inferior treatment. Attendance at out-patient clinics was also a possibility but again inferior treatment was likely. Although, according to the state of medical knowledge at the time, cures for various diseases were formulated according to individual needs, this apparently occurred only for the affluent. The 'Vagabond', a popular Victorian literary character, described treatment at the Melbourne hospital out-patient clinic as being 'rough and ready. Gallons of different medicines . . . are kept ready made up in the dispensary. What cures one will cure another seems to be the rule' (James, 1969: 26).

Little wonder than that support for unqualified practitioners was substantial. Some of this found its way into popular literature, for example in Henry Lawson's *Joe Wilson's Mate* (1970). Lawson states that he 'never had much faith in doctors', claiming he preferred his grandmother to a doctor. Later in the book he writes, 'Joe in common with most bushmen and their families round here, had more faith in Doc Weld, a weird Yankee who made medicine in a saucepan and worked more cures on bushmen than did the other three doctors of the district together' (Lawson, 1970: 174). Clearly a climate of public opinion supported unqualified practitioners. Patronage of *qualified* practitioners was discouraged furthermore through adverse press reports. The *Melbourne Punch* (18.8.1878: 4) for instance, contended that most patient deaths were the responsibility of the medical man.

The doctors' lack of success in attaining favourable legislation in the latter part of the nineteenth century can also be explained by the continuing segmentation and lack of unity. The internal disagreements which had characterised the profession in the period to 1880 continued into the 1890s. These controversies between doctors were all conducted publicly, the accusations of unprofessional conduct and replies all duly appearing in newspapers. The medical positions at Melbourne Hospital were filled by a system of elections and the touting for votes by some doctors in their public election campaigns was a source of embarrassment to the profession. As the *Melbourne Punch* (1.7.1878: 203) commented sardonically,

the fight for the hospital committeeship has extended even unto the physicians and surgeons, and medicos are at present issuing circulars by the thousand, telling our wondering little world that they, so and so, feel anxious for the vote on August the 18th next, for the delightful privilege of sawing men's limbs off or disembowelling any or everybody brought to the hospital.

James Beaney, the controversial and flamboyant surgeon of the time, openly admitted that his election to the hospital had cost him a lot of money. He also published a pamphlet entitled *Doctors Differ* which attempted to discredit the capabilities of his fellow practitioners, thus playing up differences between doctors (Craig, 1950).

The range of different professional organisations persisted furthermore. As we saw in the previous chapter, doctors in Victoria were presented by the Medical Society of Victoria (MSV) alone until 1879, when a group broke away to form the Victorian Branch of the British Medical Association (BMA). This appears to have been a reflection of the different interests of the segments which make up the medical profession. The MSV was criticised as representing only the elite of the profession and not representing the rank-and-file general practitioners. Certainly most of the leading members of the MSV were associated with the hospital or the medical school. The two organisations with some overlap of membership existed alongside each other reasonably amicably through the 1880s and 1890s, the MSV defining its role more in scientific terms and the BMA in political terms. Several attempts were made to unify the two associations but these continually foundered, partially it seems because of conflicting interests and partially because of personalities (see Pensabene, 1980: 101–106).

From the mid-1890s however the whole situation began to change as the medical elite sought to translate the legitimacy of science, claimed to be associated with the development of scientific medicine, into a market advantage. In 1891 the Melbourne Medical Association was formed comprising Melbourne graduates and this group in 1895 reestablished the Medical Defence Association (MDA), an organisation which had existed for five years from 1879 but had foundered on efforts to regulate the ethical behaviour of its members. The establishment of the MDA marks a new phase of militant professionalisation of medicine, aimed at securing the political and legislative advancement for doctors. Concern about the overcrowding in the profession which existed at the time was the immediate cause of its establishment (Pensabene, 1980: 108). However it also took on a political role in promoting and protecting doctors' interests in all areas while the other associations concentrated upon 'scientific matters'. By 1899 it had almost half the practising doctors as members and easily outstripped any of the other associations. As such it was able to provide a focus of unity. The necessity for unity as a means of achieving upward social mobility was increasingly stressed by spokesmen during this period (see IMJA, 20.6.1897: 327).

After about 1900 also the attitude in the newspapers towards doctors changed markedly from one of criticism and skepticism, to one of support and promotion (Pensabene, 1980: 40). The newspapers came to be consciously promoting practitioners of scientific medicine over other practitioners. In this favourable environment the medical elite at least were well placed socially and politically to advocate legislative enactment to secure a position of dominance for scientific medicine in the health arena.

The legislation issue was again raised in 1903 with the Medical Board pressing for a five year course as a minimum for registration. This would have the effect of regulating the supply of doctors considerably, as many parts of the world including the USA had only three year training periods. When the legislation was favourably received, further and much more radical amendments were introduced which aimed to end competition in the medical market place altogether by banning unqualified practitioners (CSO, 05/V6560, 15.11.1905). The Medical Board also pressed for much greater regulatory powers, both externally to have the right to undertake its own prosecutions (which had been vested in the Chief Secretary), as well as internally in the form of an infamous conduct clause to control the members of the profession itself. It wanted the right to strike a person off the medical register for 'infamous conduct in a professional or other respect' (CSO, 05/W6529, 14.11.1905). The government proposed to introduce felony or misdemeanour as the grounds for being struck off, but the profession revealed that the infamous conduct clause was desired specifically to stop 'covering', whereby an unqualified practitioner was employed by a qualified one to do some of this or her work (CSO, 05/W6364, 1.11.1905).

The amendments were particularly aimed at achieving control over homeopaths, whose three year (American) training would have disqualified any new homeopathic practitioners from commencing practice in Victoria. Without new practitioners, this mode of healing and the hospital utilising it could not survive. Homeopaths vehemently opposed the legislation, pressing for amendment to the legislation so that the five year training clause should not apply to homeopathic practitioners. The homeopaths drew an analogy with the principle of religious freedom in support of their arguments (CSO, 05/X6622, 2.8.1906). Herbalists also objected to the bill in libertarian ideological terms, arguing that the ban on unqualified practice 'interferes with the liberties of the public in requiring attendance with a doctor and a certain theory of medicine thereby entailed' (CSO, 05/W6529, 15.11.1905).

The government's objection to the bill, in particular the infamous conduct clause can be seen from a meeting of the Chief Secretary Sir Samuel Gillot with a joint deputation from the BMA, MDA and MMA. Gillot claimed the clause was far too wide, accorded too much power to medicine itself, and that no precedents existed. A ban on unqualified practice furthermore would rob some rural areas of any medical treatment at all. The bill was finally passed in 1908 with a number of amendments. Five years of study 'in a *regular* course of medical and surgical study' (emphasis added) was required before registration, but a compromise on the homeopaths' claim allowed only *one* new homeopathic practitioner per year from the United States to be registered. Unqualified practice was not banned, nor was 'infamous conduct' granted as grounds for action by the Medical Board (though felony and misdemeanour were).

The 1908 Act represented a major victory for scientific medicine, ensuring a position of dominance within the health arena. Foreign registration was effectively ended and the supply of doctors more easily regulated, a factor which made later unified industrial action much easier. Homeopathy and other modes of medicine were effectively controlled, indeed the passing of the Act marked the beginning of the end of homeopathy. The Medical Board gained partial autonomy and could act in cases of felony or misdemeanour, though the infamous conduct clause was not achieved until later. The 1908 Act then is important in the rise of the medical profession to the position of dominance.

State patronage of medicine had been relatively perfunctory until 1908. With internal divisions making for disunity, and general lack of effectiveness in their treatment, allopaths had been unable to distinguish themselves other than in social terms from their competitors such as homeopaths. After 1908 however the situation changed dramatically as much greater state patronage ensued for what had become the practitioners of scientific medicine. The important point (for now) about this process is that this state patronage was established in the absence of clear evidence that the practical success of the new medical technology was sufficient to bring about the scientific revolution which had occurred. While the development of the new medical technology was a necessary condition for the creation of dominance within the health arena, it was not a sufficient condition. Rather, as Kuhn argues, such 'scientific revolutions' are normally effected at the political level. Certainly the political practices of the doctors themselves were important in achieving this state patronage (ie the internal dynamic), but a consideration of the external dynamic is also important as the latter part of this chapter will elaborate.

The consolidation of medical dominance 1908–1933

The legislation of 1908 accorded much greater patronage to medicine than had previously been the case. Medical dominance however was not 'produced' fully until further legislation in 1933. The period 1908–33 is marked by the consolidation of the position of medicine. The 1908 legislation gave it considerable legal advantages; the period now to be considered sees the translation of that legal advantage into market advantage. The legal framework established in 1908 provided the basis upon which the professionalisation of medicine could proceed and its dominance could be consolidated. As previously it is useful to analyse the process in two parts, the internal and external dynamics of professionalisation.

The internal dynamic was constituted by the active pursuit of professionalisation. There were attempts to be better organised and more unified than had been the case previously. The existence of supportive legislation and a more secure technology of medical work facilitated this. There were calls for the unification of the various associations representing doctors. With favourable legislation in the pipeline, the amalgamation between the BMA (Victorian Branch) and the MSV was achieved at the end of 1906. The new body became the BMA (Vic) with about half the practitioners in the state as members. Its first task was seen as increasing membership substantially as a means of gaining much greater control over the provision of medical services in Victoria. It also attempted to unify the remaining associations, particularly the MDA. Classic strategies of professionalisation were followed such as the adoption of a national code of ethics in 1912 after the formation of a federal BMA.

Disputes between practitioners were institutionalised in the sense that procedures were set up so that these could be resolved internal to the profession. The decision was also taken at this time to stop airing its dirty linen in public by ceasing to publicise details of disputes. The code of ethics also forbade both advertising and consultation with 'irregulars' such as homeopaths. A 'black list' of practitioners who broke these ethical guidelines was instituted and this came to exert powerful social control upon members. Regional divisions were also set up and by 1913 these existed in the Goulburn Valley, the Wimmera and the western portion of the state. In 1920 students also began to be trained in medical ethics and etiquette.

The efforts directed at unifying medicine were a necessary precondition for the other major professionalisation thrust aimed at establishing control over conditions of practice and thereby greater autonomy. The attempt to replace a 'mediated' mode of control over work with one involving 'professionalism' (Johnson, 1972) occurred in the period 1910–1925 in Victoria in the struggle with the friendly societies. As employees of the friendly societies, doctors experienced a mediated work situation, and one in which their autonomy was limited. By overcoming the friendly societies doctors eliminated the major alternative entrepreneur of medical care and were thereby able to take over that role themselves and control their work situation on a more individualised fee-for-service basis (ie professionalism). The struggle with the friendly societies was therefore an important feature of the rise of medicine to political and economic power. Indeed it represented the first occasion when the profession exercised its political muscles and provided the basis for further political campaigns later in the twentieth century.

A recent analysis of this struggle has been carried out in considerable detail by Pensabene (1980: 147–158) and I propose to draw briefly upon his account. The establishment of friendly societies in Victoria was a feature of the transplantation of the English model of health and welfare services in the colonies. Friendly societies originated in England around the seventeenth century and their growth was greatly encouraged by the industrial revolution and the emergence of an industrial workforce. They were encouraged by the British government as 'self-help' societies thus absolving the state of responsibility of caring for the sick and needy. They were transplanted into the Victorian context early in the development of the colony and dominated the health scene until the emergence of the Victorian Natives Association (which only the Australian-born could join) from 1871. The societies developed as the main source of medical services for the working class in the late nineteenth century.

The medical profession initially favoured the societies, both in term of the profession's class attitudes (they promoted thrift and self-reliance among the working class) and also because they provided a source of income unattainable from private practice, as most workers could not afford private consultations. The societies also reduced the numbers attending free out-patient clinics of hospitals. The members contributed a monthly amount and the societies in return paid a doctor a capitation fee (ie an amount of money per head of population who belonged) to provide medical services for them. Society membership grew rapidly during the boom economic conditions of the 1880s, after slow growth until that time. Pensabene argues that between 1880 and 1890 total society membership doubled and there was a jump in the percentage of the total population insured with the societies from 15.1 per cent to 21.8 per cent. Doctors' dissatisfaction with what became known as the 'lodge' system, however, first expressed in 1862 (Graham, 1952: 235), gradually increased. A survey of doctors conducted by the MDA in 1898 found that 89 per cent of those who responded were unhappy with their lodge contracts (IMJA, 20.11.1889: 678). Doctors objected to their terms and conditions of work with the societies. They were in effect employees and were required to tender for contracts and patients.

There was also objection during the 1880s to the large numbers of middle class people joining the societies, thus robbing the doctors of a source of private income. Doctors objected furthermore to what they considered low remuneration for their services from the lodge and also to the wide variation in the amount paid as capitation fee.

Although dissatisfaction with lodge contracts was growing throughout the later part of the nineteenth century and early twentieth century, the doctors for a long time during this period lacked the political organisation to oppose the societies. The societies on the other hand were highly organised and unified in their dealings with the doctors. Factors which have already been discussed such as internal disunity amongst doctors and public disagreements were important in explaining this industrial weakness. However Pensabene (1980: 74) argues that also important was the fact that the number of doctors was rising faster than the population as a whole.

Indeed the recognition of the need for unity was a major factor in the unification of the various medical associations and the profession as a whole. (see Worrall, 1909: 598). From 1910, the profession began to act in more unified fashion. The amalgamation of the associations in 1907 combined with changes in the supply of doctors to improve the industrial strength of the profession. The legislative changes of 1908 had restricted the right of entry of medical immigrants, and changes in the British health system in 1911 meant a sharp decline in the number of British doctors emigrating in Victoria. The dispute got underway in earnest late in 1913. The BMA wanted an income input imposed on those who could join and a rise in the capitation fees paid.

In January, 1918, after a halt in the dispute during the early part of the First World War, most doctors resigned from the friendly societies on the instructions of the BMA, and suggested a new agreement under which they would agree to be re-employed. State government intervention followed but was unsuccessful in settling the dispute.

Finally a Royal Commission was appointed and delivered its decision in June 1918. It accepted the doctors' claim for both an income limit, (though set a higher figure than the BMA had wanted) and an increase in fees. The dispute remained deadlocked for a further eighteen months until 1920 when financial difficulties and falling membership caused the societies to give in. The medical profession had achieved its aim of the right to control the conditions of medical practice, and established fee-for-service as the mode of medical treatment henceforth.

This winning of the right to control the terms and conditions of practice is an important element in the rise of the medical profession to political and economic power. In economic terms it represented gaining control over the demand for medical services in the medical market place. Controlling the major alternative entrepreneur of

medical care, doctors established themselves firmly into a petit bourgeois entrepreneurial role. The establishment of fee-for-service as the
financial basis for medical practice was crucial in the attainment of
professionalism as the form of work control under which medical
practice was carried out in Victoria. The struggle with the friendly
societies had other consequences as well; in particular it unified
medicine much more than previously and helped contain the segmentation which had earlier characterised the profession. By the early
1920s for instance, 80 per cent of all doctors were members of the
BMA (Pensabene, 1980: 115).

The unity in opposing friendly societies proved only a temporary
one however as the segmentation between general practitioners and
specialists began to influence BMA politics. This segmentation is
today a major feature of medical politics. Its origins, it is important to
note, lie however in the period *before* the 'scientific' basis of medicine
had been clearly established. This point is important and conventional
technological determinist explanations for the growth of specialisms
(the explosion of medical knowledge) are in that sense ahistorical,
since specialists appeared in the period prior to the widespread acceptance of the germ theory of disease. As in other respects, medical
developments in Victoria followed those in the United Kingdom,
where the emergence of specialisms in the mid-Victoria era has been
analysed by Peterson (1978). Medical specialisms she argues, cannot
be explained by technical innovation or the desire for research. Rather
they were more related to survival and ambition as a form of entrepreneurial behaviour as medicine became transformed into a business
activity. The career benefits from this form of medical individualism
were not so much related to income only but also reputation building
in terms of connections and visibility (Peterson, 1978: 248–267; see
also Parry and Parry, 1976: 140).

In the period prior to 1880 furthermore it was generally not the elite
of the profession who became specialists and founded specialist institutions. The development of specialties, Peterson argues, was a
feature of the growth in medical individualism (as was patent
medicines) which the elite of the profession was attempting to control
and regulate through collectivist occupational associations. Such
individualism, as Larson (1977) has argued, was only possible in an
occupation without a secure knowledge base.

By 1920 however various specialties had begun to appear, surgery
being one of the first. In 1926 the Australian College of Surgeons was
established, outside the BMA. This led to an outcry from members of
the BMA, especially from the general practitioners. The dispute came
to a head in 1930 when a motion was successfully moved in the BMA
that the college of surgeons was 'inimical to the best interests of the
members of this branch' (MJA, 21.4.1928: 504). A battle for control

of the profession ensued which was won by the general practitioner section and the major threat to the unity of the BMA was contained.

As well as controlling the demand for medical services, medicine also moved during this period to control the supply of practitioners both 'unqualified' and 'qualified'. The 1908 legislation restricted eligibility for registration to those countries which allowed reciprocal registration. Only New Zealand, Canada, Britain and Italy had such arrangements. Medicine also continued its campaign to remove unqualified or 'irregular' practitioners and thus control competition within the medical marketplace. As we have seen, prior to 1900 their attempts met with relatively little success. After 1900 however the situation was different.

The 1908 Act gave medicine considerable legislative advantages which they then set about translating into market advantages. The development of chemotherapy, a change in the role of hospitals from being just charitable institutions to caring for all the sick on a fee-paying basis, and greater unity within medical profession, all combined to decrease support for unqualified practitioners. Indeed the number of unqualified practitioners declined during this time—the number describing themselves as 'irregular medical practitioners' in the census declined by over 40 per cent between 1911 and 1921.

This process was aided by editorial opinion in the newspapers. Indeed *The Argus* published several articles supporting the suppression of unqualified practitioners:

> All that can be said for the quack remedies even at their best is that they may be harmless. At their worst they are extremely dangerous ... Any means that can decrease quackery will be welcome ... the real science of medicine has made wonderful advances and medicine at its best is fully represented in Victoria by men of the highest qualifications obtainable and the best knowledge. (The Argus, 27.4.1925: 10)

The major competitors to medicine however were homeopaths and the demise of homeopathy was essential to the dominance of medicine within the health arena. A major blow to homeopathy, as we have seen, was the clause in the 1908 medical Act which restricted the registration of new homeopathic practitioners to just one per year. This, as expected, resulted in difficulties in staffing the homeopathic hospital. There were also ideological disagreements amongst hospital practitioners between the 'straights' who practised solely homeopathic techniques and the 'mixers' who combined homeopathic and allopathic techniques, attempting to take the best from both. The code of ethics passed by the BMA in 1912 had a clause specifically forbidding members to consult with a homeopath in treatment and threatening to blacklist any member who did so. All these factors, along with a growing support for the germ theory of disease, contributed to the demise of homeopathy (Templeton, 1969; Pensabene, 1980: 133-139).

Finally in the 1920s the BMA adopted a takeover policy towards the homeopathic hospital. It decided not to enforce the ethical requirement of non-consultation with homeopaths so that its members could accept appointments at the hospital. Faced with an inability to appoint sufficient homeopathic practitioners to staff the hospital, the management had little choice but to appoint BMA members. More and more gradually came to practise at the hospital, and this combined with financial difficulties engendered by the depression of the 1930s led to a decision in 1934 to move away from a close association with homeopathy and the hospital was renamed 'Prince Henry's Hospital' (Templeton, 1969). The demise of homeopathy was complete and the source of supply of homeopathic practitioners and treatment competitive with that offered by the BMA were controlled. By the early 1930s the professionalisation of medicine was well established. Both the demand for its services and the supply of practitioners to meet that demand had been controlled.

Armed with a more secure and politically useful technology of work, doctors were also to successfully press their claims for autonomy and dominance within the health sector. A major success was achieved in 1908 as we have seen but was not finally achieved until 1933. It remains to analyse briefly the legislative changes in the period 1908-1933.

As we have seen, the medical profession pressed for the inclusion of an 'infamous conduct' clause as grounds for deregistration by the Medical Board from early in the period. They were denied it in 1908 and its achievement was a major aim between then and 1933 when it was finally established. During the period however further advances were made in securing legislative advantage. In 1915 for instance the use of the term 'doctor' was restricted to those registered under the Act. By 1933, Victoria was the only state in the Commonwealth which did not have an 'infamous conduct' clause and the legislation was precipitated by reports that a doctor, struck off the medical register in NSW, was about to settle in Victoria where registration could not legally be denied him (VPD, 27.7.1933: 575). The legislation was also introduced as a means of bolstering trust in the medical profession as a matter of public interest. As Dr Shields, one of the medically qualified members of the legislature claimed, the legislation was needed because 'You must retain the confidence of the public in the medical profession' (VPD, 23.8.1933: 1003). The government under its premier Sir Stanley Argyle (also medically qualified) was reluctant to define 'infamous conduct', preferring to give the Medical Board wide powers, but when pressed admitted seduction of 'household members' and drunkenness (and not political offences) were the intended grounds. The bill however generated little opposition, and had the easiest passage through parliament of any of the medical bills of the period. By gaining such legislation the profession was able to supervise the professional behaviour of its members without recourse to authority outside the profession itself. The essential condition for autonomy and thereby professionalism as a mode of control over work had been established. The 'production' of medical dominance was also completed.

Medical training and the class compatibility of knowledge

Having analysed the process of professionalisation, the importance of the development of scientific knowledge can be seen. Yet while it was important, it must be seen as only one of the resources available to medicine in the political process. The production of medical dominance was primarily a political process in which the scientific knowledge was part, as were other aspects such as the claim to effectiveness. A transition in paradigms of medical knowledge and the technology of medical work occurred as scientific medicine was introduced. This new paradigm was qualitatively different from (ie only partially commensurable with) that utilised by allopaths previously. This group utilised the growing legitimacy of science as a means of collective upward social mobility. Such advancement was only possible as state patronage of medicine grew to a point of legally sustained and created dominance within the health arena.

Yet this state patronage was achieved, I believe, in the absence of clear evidence that the practical success of the new technology was sufficient to bring about the scientific revolution which occurred. Most accounts attribute the success of medicine to the nature of the new technology itself. The development of the new technology I believe to be a necessary but not a sufficient condition for the production of medical dominance. Medicine claimed the legitimacy of science and its effectiveness as a means of collective self advancement; as Kuhn has argued, scientific revolutions are effected at the political level by the political practices of (in this case) doctors. Yet also important in explaining the production of medical dominance is the external dynamic of professionalisation, of which technological determinist explanations insufficiently take account. Such an external dynamic is constituted by the political economy of Australian society and the class relationships which form an integral part of that political economy.

A distinct aspect of the political process of the production of medical dominance is the compatibility of the mode of medical knowledge with dominant class ideologies. In what follows I will attempt to demonstrate how this applies to the development of medical training and research. This is a key area in which to examine the political processes involved since a new paradigm is progressively established through its transmission and inculcation (together with ideological elements) into new entrants to the occupation. 'Scientific' medicine was gradually introduced into the training institution of the medical profession in Victoria (the Melbourne University Medical School) over the period under consideration.

First however it is necessary to examine the issue of 'compatibility' and its applicability to the Australian context. To do this involves articulating the relationship between changes in medical knowledge and technology and class interests outlined briefly in a previous chapter. This has been done for the American context by Berliner (1975, 1977) and Brown (1979). Berliner documents how the 'progressive era' in the United States around the turn of the century was characterised by the development of science in all fields of human endeavour including management (Taylorism), agriculture, social work, motherhood and 'domestic science', and most importantly medicine. This development, which as Larson and others have argued was a major feature in the structural transformation of the economy from laissez-faire to monopoly capitalism, was also felt in Australia as Michael Roe (1977) has shown. However Berliner goes on to discuss how this appeal to science—what he calls scientism—became an important form of authority and social control, masked by the name of science, mediated through middle class professional organisations but supported and funded by upper class groups.

In the medical sphere, Berliner argues, 'scientific medicine' was the name usurped by the allopathic sect in their struggle against opposing modes such as homeopathy. But it was the ideological assumptions which underlie scientific medicine which led to strong dominant class support for the germ theory or scientific medicine, and hence for its practitioners, allopaths. Scientific medicine was based on the ideological assumption that disease was an individual and a biological phenomenon, rather than a social and environmental one as some theories in the 1850s in Europe had claimed. Berliner's prime focus is on the role of the philanthropic foundations such as the Rockefeller and Carnegie foundations in promoting such a paradigm. According to Berliner, the main advisor to the Rockefellers on medical matters (Gates) quickly realised the advantages of such a paradigm, saying that 'people were not unhealthy because of the system and relations of production they lived under, but rather because of germs which would be eliminated' (Berliner, 1977: 107).

By defining ill-health as a scientific problem, only technical and technological solutions were required, whereas defining it as a social problem demanded political solutions. 'Rather than making the reasonable assumption that while bacteria were the prime causative agents of disease, their pathogenic effects on the body being mediated socially and environmentally, physicians of the time totally dismissed social and environmental factors in the conventional understanding of the germ theory' (Berliner, 1977: 103).

None of this implies a conspiracy theory it should be noted. Rather the argument that Berliner makes is of the compatibility of the germ theory with dominant class interests, a factor which led to the activities of the foundations in reforming medical education in the United States so as to promote 'scientific medicine'. When we come to examine the applicability of Berliner's thesis in the Victorian context there is some evidence at least of support from business interests for scientific medicine from about 1900.

One area where this can be seen is in newspaper editorials which I would argue following Gramsci are an important aspect in the maintenance of ideological hegemony in capitalist societies. As Pensabene has shown (though uses for a different argument), editorials in Melbourne newspapers, particularly *The Argus* which had frequently been critical prior to 1900, after that date began to promote scientific medicine. In 1911 for instance it argued that 'the medical man of today is essentially a healer and that means a peculiar combination of scientist, priest and teacher, combined with firm nerve and great skill of hand' (The Argus, 16.9.1911: 18). By 1912, it was quoting Robert Louis Stevenson:

There are men and classes of men that stand above the common herd; the soldier, the sailor and the shepherd not infrequently; the artist rarely, the clergyman rarer still; the physician almost as a rule. He is the flower (such as it is) of our civilisation and when that stage of man is done with, he will be thought to have shared as little as any in the defects of the period, and most noticeably exhibited the virtues of the race. (The Argus, 17.8.1912: 12)

The other area where class interests were involved was in medical education, and it is now possible to analyse the introduction of scientific medicine into the Melbourne Medical School in some detail. This process has been analysed by Russell (1977) in his book *The Melbourne Medical School, 1862–1962*.

Firstly it should be noted that because of the distance of Australia from the centres of discovery and innovation in Europe during this period, an important feature of the changes in medical education were various trips made by prominent medical school academics to study and evaluate developments in medicine and medical education, and to evaluate the feasibility of introducing these developments into the curriculum. In this of course, Victoria was following changes already occurring in the northern hemisphere as the new paradigm spread thoughout the industrialising capitalist world. Journeys were made to Europe in 1881, 1890 and 1912, and to the United States in 1927. The last mentioned journey is significant as American influence on medical education began to assert itself. Each of these trips was followed by a report showing how teaching at the Melbourne Medical School lagged behind developments in overseas education and calling for curriculum changes. These changes were often not introduced for several years, mainly because the University Council claimed inability to meet the additional financial expenditure the modifications would require.

The curriculum was modified on five occasions as inculcation of the new paradigm was gradually established. Following his European trip in 1881 the Dean, George Britton Halford, together with another staff member Harry Brookes Allen, recommended substantial curriculum changes. Less emphasis was to be placed on 'pure' science subjects such as physics and more on subjects central to the new medical technology such as practical physiology (Russell, 1977: 13) though it took until 1906 before all the recommendations were introduced. Allen travelled to Europe in 1890 'to catch up on developments in scientific medicine' and his report advocated more emphasis on the 'new medical sciences' (such as histology and histopathology) which were emerging with the development of the germ theory. In 1899 the curriculum was 'modernised' as Russell (1977: 90) describes it, as instruction in the new 'specialisms' such as gynaecology and diseases of the eye, skin etc, commenced. Also from about 1900 medical research began in a systematic way in Victoria and gradually assumed more importance.

In 1904, concern over the adequacy of the socialisation of medical students resulted in a Royal Commission into medical education. More instruction in science subjects such as physiology and biology was recommended along with the increase in the amount of clinical training which Halford had recommended and on which he had been opposed in 1890. Russell argues that the modern day curriculum (with a few modifications) dates from 1911. The recognition of hospitals as clinical schools dates from this time as well.

The other major change occurred in 1923, following a meeting of representatives of all Australian medical schools in 1920, at which it was decided to increase the length of training, the extra two terms to be a basic first year course in physics, chemistry and biology. Fees were also increased by 20 per cent (Russell, 1977: 130–131). The change was spurred in major part by concern with 'overcrowding' within the profession and a desire to reduce the numbers of new entrants. This went along with efforts to control the supply of all practitioners detailed previously, and was aimed at making quality medical care into a scarcer commodity to strengthen the position of doctors in all respects, financially, socially and politically.

The number of students at the Melbourne Medical School had grown only slowly until 1900. This appears to have been a result of a high failure rate (50 per cent in 1884) (AMJ, 15.12.1884: 555–558) and the tendency for some students to complete their degrees overseas, particularly in the United Kingdom, after completing the first year course at Melbourne. In his analysis of obituary notices appearing in the *Medical Journal of Australia* (MJA) between 1921 and 1930, Pensabene (1980: 64) counted 30 doctors who had done this, of whom twenty had attended Edinburgh University. After 1900, however, the number of medical students expanded rapidly (Russell, 1977: 218–219).

The boom period of the 1880s led to the development of a 'colonial bourgeoisie' (Dickey, 1974) and the medical profession represented an attractive career for the sons of this class. The first women medical students began training in 1887 as well (Russell, 1977: 74–77). Other middle class groups such as teachers and accountants also aspired to their offspring gaining upward social mobility through education. For the working class however, entry into medicine was almost impossible. The prerequisites of classical learning in Latin and Greek which mainly private schools taught, made entry into medical school extremely difficult even without considering tuition fees payable to the university. In his analysis of obituary notices mentioned above, Pensabene (1980: 74) found that only 21 per cent of the doctors whose obituary notices appeared in the MJA between 1921 and 1930, had been to state high schools, and only nine per cent had been to Catholic schools. Students from Protestant private schools dominated the profession. This meant that recruitment was class restrictive: almost 45 per cent of these doctors came from families where the father was involved in one of three occupations: doctors, clergymen and graziers (Pensabene, 1980: 70). No working class occupations were represented, the nearest being a court clerk. This is not surprising when it is considered that in 1904 for example the average weekly wage in manufacturing was £1–15–0 (£91 pa) (MacCarthy, 1970: 56–76); while the yearly fees in the medical school, exclusive of the cost of text and notebooks was more than double that of £184–16–0 (Melbourne University Calendar, 1904).

After World War I the number of students entering Melbourne Medical School had increased dramatically, as it did at Sydney and Adelaide. Considerable overcrowding resulted and in this context members of the three faculties met in 1920 to discuss control over numbers and the curriculum change outlined above was the result. It was introduced in 1923 and immediately had the desired effect. In 1924 the intake was only 65, the lowest since 1900 and down from 202 in 1920 (Pensabene, 1980: 72). The major consequence of the changes from a social and political viewpoint was to make entry into medicine even more class restrictive. Higher fees and a longer period of training before an income could be earned, restricted even further the class background from which medical students originated. Whether this was an intended or unintended consequence is not entirely clear but the decision to reduce the numbers by this rather than some other method does seem to indicate awareness of the class restrictive nature of the changes.

The other major area where class interests were involved in the introduction of the new medical knowledge was in corporate sponsorship, medical education and research. In Berliner's study the prime focus is on the involvement of the philanthropic foundations in the establishment of the paradigm of scientific medicine. This involvement saw the sponsoring of the Flexner report, a study of medical education in the early twentieth century which led to its reform in the direction of the teaching of scientific medicine. This reform was paid for by the foundations themselves. Thus Berliner (1975) argues, the corporate class in the United States was important in promoting a paradigm of medicine which was compatible with their interests. This is not to imply the germ theory was a creation of powerful economic interests, but that their support and encouragement aided and speeded its introduction into medical schools and facilitated the rise of the medical profession to political and economic power. By providing endowments and financial support, the introduction of scientific medicine was achieved much faster than if financial support had not been forthcoming.

Evidence of the involvement of national and international capital in the development of the Melbourne Medical School can be seen from an examination of benefactions received. The first benefaction the Melbourne Medical School received was in 1981 when the controversial local practitioner, James Beaney, gave £3900 for scholarships in surgery and pathology (List of Principal Benefactions, 1959). A number of medical practitioners gave donations during the period but from 1900 benefactions from business sources began to appear. Amongst the benefactors some leading industrialists of the time are represented. The David Syme Charitable Trust, created by the owner of *The Age* newspaper, gave £3000 for scientific research in 1904, and £500 for equipment in 1913. Geelong chemical manufacturer, Richard Fletcher, gave £7500 for cancer and anaesthetics research in 1926 and £4960 for medical research in 1930. However amongst the promoters of scientific medicine one name appears consistently—that of Edward Wilson, owner of *The Argus* newspaper. Large sums of money flowed from the trust set up by him to donate money after his death in 1878. In 1907, £100,000 was offered by the trustees to Melbourne Hospital to rebuild; in 1925, £9206 was given to Melbourne Medical School for obstetrical research; in 1919, £20,000 was given to establish a chair of obstetrics; £900 was given in 1925 for psychiatric research; £400 in

1927 for cancer research; £400 in 1929 for gastric research (List of Principal Benefactions, 1959).

Besides these local capitalists there was also promotion from international capital, indeed from the very philanthropic foundations which Berliner has examined, through their international aid programme. One of the issues which dominated the development of medical services and medical education was the long controversy over the re-siting of Melbourne Hospital. With the advent of scientific medicine with its bulky technology such as X-ray machines, and the growing emphasis on clinical training for medical students, a decision to rebuild the Melbourne Hospital (which had been built in 1848) was inevitable. However controversy raged over many years as to whether the hospital should be rebuilt on its existing site or on a new site. The promise of a large donation from the Edward Wilson Trust in 1907, provided the hospital was rebuilt on its present site, was ajudged too good to refuse despite the opposition of the medical faculty who wanted the hospital located on another site (its present-day one) closer to the medical school (Inglis, 1958; Russell, 1977: 112–113).

By 1913 the hospital had been rebuilt, temporarily as it later turned out. In 1914 Berry, a leading member of the medical faculty who was later to become dean submitted his 'Plan for the Consolidation of Scientific Medicine' (Medical Faculty Minutes, 1914). This 'bold, enlightened and very practical' scheme as Russell (1977: 113) describes it, suggested that the medical school be relocated in the hospital grounds in a new large building thus reflecting the growing emphasis on clinical training in medical education. His plan received approval from the profession and the hospital but the unavailability of finance due to the outbreak of the war was the response of the government.

During the 1920s, however, when the question of the move of the hospital to the Parkville site again became a possibility, the faculty wrote in 1923 to the Rockefeller Foundation in the United States for financial assistance in relocating. The foundation responded in a letter indicating they would send their associate director of the division of medical education, 'to familiarise himself with medical education here' (Medical Faculty Minutes, 1923). The faculty resolved to pursue this in an attempt to attract endowment and supplied the further information the foundation requested. The Rockefeller representative duly visited Melbourne in May 1924 and was shown over the facilities and furnished with the information he required. He appears to have caused some consternation amongst faculty members by arriving unannounced and looking around himself before revealing he was the foundation's representative. In 1926 the faculty minutes record the decision of the Victorian government to relocate the medical school itself and the interest of the foundation appears to have changed. Shortly after an invitation was issued from the foundation for someone from the medical school to come to the United States 'as a guest of the foundation, to inspect the most up-to-date medical institutions' (Medical Faculty Minutes, 1926). The all-expenses-paid visit by Berry, mentioned earlier was the result in 1927, his report being presented to the faculty in 1928.

More information on why the Rockefeller Foundation decided not to endow the Melbourne Medical School at this time is available from the in-house history of the foundation by Fosdick (1952: 109–122). One important element of the reform of medical education which the foundation was promoting was its 'full-time clinical plan'. The aim was to have professors of clinical medicine paid fixed salaries and not have the right to private practice. This was considered essential to encourage research as the professor would spend his entire time devoted to research and teaching and not to private practice which would otherwise have limited his time for research. The English medical education system after which the Victorian was modelled, guaranteed the right of private practice for medical school staff though this was a frequent source of conflict between the medical faculty and the university administration in the development of the medical school, as Russell indicates. While the Rockefeller Foundation were quite successful in achieving this in the United States, they were much less successful in Britain and in Australia. What Fosdick (1952: 90) argues is that while the foundation was considering its response to the Melbourne University request, they saw an opportunity to promote their full-time plan elsewhere in Australia as 'a promising apportunity developed at the University of Sydney where a local citizen has recently given large sums towards the establishment of several full-time chairs'.

The foundation gave £100,000 towards the cost of building and equipping clinical laboratories at the University of Sydney in the belief, according to Fosdick (1952: 135), quoting Rockefeller Foundation minutes, that it would 'produce in Australia, decided results, both in the way of an admirable school and an influence in the dominion'. Thus they appear to have operated a 'regional' concept. By endowing one school in the country (Sydney) they hoped it would become an example which other medical schools, such as Melbourne, would attempt to emulate.

The local capitalist in Sydney was George Henry Bosch, who before he gave the gift of £225,000 to establish the chairs of Medicine, Surgery and Bacteriology, 'took the trouble to make a thorough study of the needs of modern medicine and how they were being met elsewhere before he made his munificent gift' (Sydney Morning Herald, 29.8.1933). At the opening of the Rockefeller funded building which coincided with the 50th Jubilee of the Sydney Medical School, the Governor of New South Wales, Sir Phillip Woolcott Game, indicated the degree of acceptance of the full-time clinical plan. Commenting on the growth in medical research, he said: 'In still more recent times, many medical centres have come to realise that, if medicine and surgery are to progress, they too must take their place within the Faculty as scientific departments equipped with adequate laboratories and with staffs whose entire activities are devoted to the work of their departments' (Pamphlet—The University of Sydney Jubilee of Medical School 1883–1933).

That the full-time plan was pressed, often against the wishes of the petit-bourgeois businessmen/doctors, is indicated by the controversy over the establishment of the new chair of obstetrics at Melbourne University in 1928 (Medical Faculty Minutes, 1928). The University Council wanted the position to be filled on a full-time basis, whereas the faculty wanted the right of private practice retained. A sub-committee was formed to resolve the issue but further controversy ensued when the two medical representatives refused to sign the report; but in 1929 it became the first full-time clinical chair.

The involvement of the Rockefeller Foundation in the Melbourne Medical School does not end here however. When the decision was finally taken by the Victorian government to move the hospital to the (present) Parkville site in 1935, a further request for endowment was made to the foundation to assist in the construction of new buildings (Russell, 1977: 156). Again, as in 1924 an offer of an all-expenses-paid trip to the United States to investigate developments in medical education was made by the foundation in 1935, and Professor MacCallum went on a seven week trip (Medical Faculty Minutes, 1935). Apparently the regional concept was still in operation, for money was not forthcoming at that time either. However, it was finally in 1960 when £50,000 was donated, again in conjunction with local endowments (of £150,000 from Myer retailing and Potter share-broking interests) for the construction of experimental laboratories in physiology (Russell, 1977: 200).

Thus business interests, both national and international, were involved in promoting the paradigm of scientific medicine in Victoria. Their involvement furthermore was specifically directed towards certain sorts of developments, in particular the new 'hard science' departments such as physiology, histology and bacteriology where germ theory research was carried out. These developments were promoted rather than departments of social medicine or community health. Endowment of research and the promotion of the full-time clinical plan which was associated with the research was important in the development of the new paradigm. Endowments for specific projects helped to define exactly what scientific medicine was going to mean and where major developments were likely to occur. Support for the germ theory placed responsibility for disease on an individual and amoral microbe rather than the environment (as the miasmatic theory had) or the social relations of production (as social medicine had). While the money donated probably did not constitute a major source of funding for the medical school, it does indicate a general affinity between bourgeois interests and scientific medicine. Germ theory in other words was attuned to the interests of the dominant class. As it developed it became consistent with and defensive of a growing capitalist economy (see Berliner, 1977: 107–108).

Such an affinity I believe is necessary in explaining the development of state patronage for medicine and the role of class interests in the professionalisation of medicine. Again as Berliner (1977: 145) argues in relation to the Flexner report in the United States, 'the changes in education and professional education that the Carnegie Foundation sponsored were serious, ideologically important, reforms of the social structure'. They were important he argues, because of the foundation's belief in the socially ameliorative qualities of education in assuaging class tensions (the Carnegie Foundation even gave some £6000 between 1904 and 1937 to Melbourne University for adult education), the perceived need for a highly skilled labour force to administer the new technology of medicine, and as a conscious attempt by the Carnegie Foundation to build up professional groups. These groups would act both as a buffer between the capitalists and the workers and also foster dependency on the part of the working class, in different areas of life (such as health, law, etc) where they were being ministered to by experts who were outside their class domain. Thus Berliner argues,

> the Carnegie Foundation saw a part of its function as creating or fostering a growing dependence of the working class on a newly resurrected petit-bourgeois professional strata ... As science was the keyword of the period, using the aura of science was a way of being able of redefine professions to change them to suit the needs of the capitalist class. (1977: 100)

The changes in medical education associated with the introduction of scientific medicine thus had two effects: one was to fully incorporate medical research into the nature of medical education (through the full-time clinical plan), the other as we have seen was to change the class composition of medical students.

Contrary to technological determinist arguments then, I wish to argue that the dominance of scientific medicine over other forms of medical knowledge, and also the hegemony of the practitioners of that knowledge over the practitioners of other modes of medical knowledge, is based upon this relationship of compatibility. To view professionalisation just as a result of the actions of the medical profession itself, without a consideration of the wider context, is only half the story. In explaining the phenomenon of medical dominance more importantly, it is the minor half. As Johnson (1977: 98) has argued, the focus cannot be on the social division of labour alone, but instead must be on the way in which this social division of labour is conditioned by the surplus value-producing processes of capital. Professionalism, the self governing mode of work control to which doctors were aspiring, and had achieved by the end of the period under consideration, arises when the political and economic conditions necessary to sustain it coincide with the interests of the dominant class. As Navarro (1976: 14) argues, 'the medical profession is a stratum of trustworthy representatives to whom the bourgeoisie delegates some of its authority to run the house of medicine'. This occurred in Victoria, I would argue, in the period after 1900.

Medical dominance was thus achieved by 1933. The development of scientific medicine, by the complex process outlined, facilitated its production. Sectarian conflicts were resolved, segmentary conflicts at least contained, and a basis established whereby hierarchical relations could be established and confirmed. Contrary to technological determinist explanations of this process however, I have argued that political and social elements did not just intrude into the process of the establishment of scientific medicine. On the contrary I have attempted to show the process was basically a political one in which scientific and technological elements intruded. Foremost in the political process were class elements, involved in two respects, both directly with regard to the class backgrounds of doctors, but also indirectly in the wider politico-economic sphere. A particular paradigm of medical knowledge and technology was promoted by bourgeois interests based upon the general affinity between germ theory and bourgeois individualism.

5   The subordination of midwifery

The other 'moment' in the development of a differentiated division of labour in health care to be analysed is the reproduction of medical dominance. The previous two chapters dealt with the production of this dominance; the focus in this second part of the study will be upon the various modes of domination by which reproduction has been achieved. One health occupation will be selected to illustrate and examine each of the three modes of domination: subordination, limitation and exclusion. In each case the development of the relationship between medicine and the chosen occupation will be used to explain the operation of the corresponding mode of domination.

The mode of domination to be analysed in this chapter is subordination. The largest proportion of health occupations experience this form of domination in the sense that the content of their work is comprised of tasks delegated to them by doctors; tasks associated with treatment that are carried out largely at the direction of doctors. As a group, subordinate health occupations have several features in common, the major one of which is that they are comprised overwhelmingly of women. They work mostly in institutionalised medical settings such as hospitals and receive lower payment for their work than do doctors.

Within this large group of health workers, comprising the bulk of the health workforce, one relatively small and specialised occupation —midwifery—has been chosen to illustrate the historical process of the reproduction of medical dominance through subordination. Now a specialised branch of nursing, though formerly an independent occupation, midwifery has been chosen for two reasons. Firstly it is an occupation which until very recently (1975) has been sex-specific in that historically, only women have been legally able to practise as midwives and unless indicated the term midwife is used here to apply to female midwives. It thus allows an examination of gender as a basis for the division of labour in health care in a relatively 'pure' form. The relationship between the sexual division of labour and the occupational division of labour can thus be explored, as can the wider issue of the relative importance of gender and class as bases for the division of labour in health care.

The second reason for choosing midwifery follows from the materialist assumption on which this study is based. A discussion of the evolution of health care, it is argued, must be rooted in the political economy of the society as a whole. Midwifery thereby is a crucial occupation within the health system because it is concerned with the *reproduction of labour power* in a society. Such a concern with labour power is crucial to the reproduction of the social relations of production necessary for the continued existence of capitalism (or indeed any other mode of production). As this chapter will argue, the reproduction of labour power has been an important theme in the development of Australian capitalism, particularly in the early twentieth century. An understanding of these broader politico-economic issues is crucial in analysing the evolution of the occupation of midwifery and its relationship with medicine.

The process to be analysed is a complex one. In the simplest terms the subordination of midwives was achieved by its incorporation into nursing, an occupation which was already structurally located in a position of subordination to medicine. By becoming in effect a special branch of nursing, something the leaders of the occupation of nursing themselves encouraged as a strategy in their own attempts at professionalisation, midwifery changed its structural location within the health division of labour from an independent status to a subordinate one.

Four periods are to be analysed in tracing this process. Firstly, as with the tracing of the evolution of the medical profession, the *English antecedents* of the occupation of midwifery are traced up until the middle of the nineteenth century. Then the evolution of the occupation in Australia, and particularly in Victoria, is traced in three periods, the *Pioneer Era* until 1880, covering very early settlement including the convict era; the *Transitional Era* from 1880 until 1910, and the *Era of Takeover* from 1910 until the late 1930s when the medical takeover was completed. Of the four periods, the first three, involving the period up until about 1910, overlap with the process of the production of doctor dominance and were obviously a part of it. The major time period to be analysed therefore is that more specifically concerned with reproduction after 1910, by which time as we have seen, the dominance of doctors had been achieved in substantial part.

The process to be analysed is the changing division of labour in attending the event of childbirth or parturition. In this change, both the gender and class basis of childbirth attendance was affected, as the change has been basically from attendance by working class women to attendance by middle class men. Associated with this change in attendant has been a transition from home to hospital as the location of childbirth. Both the sexual division of labour and the occupational division of labour were thus transformed.

Two sources of complexity should be noted in this process. The first is the segmentation of both medicine and nursing. Although at first glance the struggle may appear to have been between doctors and midwives, two other sources of conflict need to be borne in mind. One is within medicine itself, between the elite who had little to do with childbirth, and who therefore were not naturally opposed to independent midwives; and the rank-and-file general practitioners for whom obstetrics was a recognised way of building up a practice. For this latter group, independent midwives were a major competitor. Further segmentation within medicine appeared also with the emergence of the specialty of obstetrics. The other source of conflict was between nursing and midwifery. In the evolution of nursing as an occupation, an attempt was made from the outset to define its occupational territory as including childbirth. The basis of this claim seems to have been that it was women who were involved in midwifery and nursing was specifically created to provide non-industrial employment for women, most of whom were middle class. A health occupation having emerged specifically for women, midwives resisted being incorporated into nursing with the subordination which that entailed.

The second source of complexity is the paucity of published material on midwives. Especially in early Australian history, midwives left few records, had no journals, wrote no accounts of their work. Whereas with doctors there is a wealth of written material this is certainly not the case with the occupation of midwifery, which appears to have had very little occupational organisation. For this reason, it has been necessary to go beyond just Victoria to examine the experience of other states as well. Oral histories have also been used and this has proved useful for the 'takeover' period after 1910. Use has been made also of accounts in the doctors' journals though as an unbiased account of the practice of midwifery they obviously have some limitations. Indeed the history of obstetrics has overwhelmingly been written by obstetricians who provide a particular 'reading' of its development. As Rich (1976: 130) argues, 'in reading the history of childbirth we have to "read between the lines" of histories of obstetrics by contemporary medical men'.

English antecedents

The occupation of midwifery is an ancient one, traditionally a non-medical lay craft practised by women until about the seventeenth century. None of the orders of medical practitioner of the time (physicians, surgeons, apothecaries) received training in midwifery, or saw pregnancy as a medical responsibility. The reason Versluysen (1981: 23) argues, drawing on a number of sources, was that midwifery was seen as 'women's work' from time immemorial. As the universities and medical corporations developed she argues, the title 'medical' gradually came to be associated with the male sex as women were progressively excluded from formal medical practice (see also Radcliffe, 1967). As a result, 'All the sources on pre-seventeenth century English midwifery confirm that it was a folk craft, and, whilst it is possible that medical men did occasionally attend births, this would have been exceptional' (Versluysen, 1981: 23).

From early in the seventeenth century however the term 'man-midwife' appears in the language and marks the beginning of a struggle between male and female midwives that was to last into the twentieth century. Indeed an early part of the strategy of male take-over was to degenderise the term 'midwife' which led to a variety of terms being used to describe males who practised midwifery. These included male-midwife, man-midwife, midman, physician man-midwife, accoucheur (rejected as being not English), even androboe-thognist (see Forbes, 1971: 354). The overwhelming proportion of deliveries in the seventeenth century continued to be carried out by midwives, according to Forbes (1971), though the popularity of male-midwives was increasing during this century. The attendance of a male-midwife at the confinement of the consort of Charles I promoted this as did the invention of the obstetrical forceps by the Chamberlens, a family of male-midwives who kept them secret and for their exclusive use and gain until the 1730s. This rather grubby piece of commercialism meant that many women and children who might otherwise have been saved, died because their birth attendant did not have access to 'the secret'. Forceps eventually came into regular usage under a male monopoly and this also contributed to the increasing appearance of men in the delivery room. By 1750, Forbes (1971: 354) estimated there were some hundreds of male-midwives in London alone and that by the latter part of the eighteen century they had gained most of the better paid midwifery work.

Most babies continued to be delivered by midwives however through the eighteenth and into the nineteenth centuries, though both Donnison and Forbes argue that the occupation of midwifery was in decline as the general practitioner gradually emerged. 'As the 18th century wore on, so the decline of the midwife continued—a cumulative process accelerated by the interested propaganda of a section of the medical profession and in particular of younger men, anxious to capture the midwifery which gave the entree to general practice' (Donnison, 1977: 37).

During the mid-eighteenth century another development occurred which formed part of the strategy of gaining professional male medical control over childbirth. After 1739, 'lying-in' hospitals began to be established by men-midwives, initially in London and later in the provinces. As Versluysen (1981: 19) argues, these hospitals 'set an important precedent in the history of childbirth since they represented the first successful attempt in this country [UK] to bring parturition under professional medical management in a secular institutional setting and provided a model for later hospital development'. The establishment of lying-in hospitals she argues cannot be explained by technical developments such as forceps, nor by improvements in medical knowledge. Instead their establishment formed part of a strategy of establishing male control over childbirth. Creating a hospital environment in which healthy working class women could give birth had a number of advantages to men-midwives. It gave them access to clinical experience and teaching material which would legitimate male medical management of childbirth. As a result their claims would be strengthened to attend births of women from other classes for which payment could be received. There was little employment for midwives within lying-in hospitals as a result, and where they were employed they could be subordinated.

The trend toward male involvement in childbirth met with vigorous opposition from midwives and a flood of polemical literature from the mid-seventeenth century demonstrates the hostility between male and female practitioners (Versluysen, 1981: 27). Opposition also came however from the elite of the profession, who considered midwifery 'the work of women and beneath the dignity of the professional man' (quoted in Donnison, 1977: 47). When a male-midwife, Sir David Hamilton was knighted in 1780, the first of his occupation to be so honoured; the couplet was published: ' "Rise up Sir David" said the Queen "the first cunt-knight that e'er was seen" ' (quoted in Stone, 1977: 73). The low status of obstetrics was confirmed by the 1858 Medical Act which did not require medical practitioners to be qualified in midwifery (indeed not till 1886 was this required), 'an omission which gave legal confirmation to the still current view that this specialty was not really part of medicine' (Donnison, 1977: 56). Men-midwives were banned from the court of assistants of the Surgeons Company for instance (Versluysen, 1981: 28–29).

An account of the position of midwifery in the mid-nineteenth century, the end of this period under consideration, is provided by Donnison (1977: 59). The majority of births she argues, were still attended by women, the exceptions being in the affluent areas of the larger cities. However the general picture at this time was one of decline:

> In some areas, midwives might attend the wives of small tradesman or farmers, but in others their clientele consisted only of the class just above paupers and here such women eked out a poor living with other humble work such as washing or charing. In some more

affluent districts they might have hardly any cases at all. (Donnison, 1977: 59)

The status of medicine on the other hand was rising as the process of professionalisation got under way. Midwives by contrast had no society and no journals, and 'most midwives had to work very long hours to make even an adequate living and few could have the education or leisure necessary to organise themselves for the improvement of the general body' (Donnison, 1977: 61). The status of the occupation had thus declined; indeed in the Victorian age with opposition to employment for middle class women, a stigma became attached to the name 'midwife', a term which could scarcely be mentioned in polite company as it alluded to matters associated with sexuality and reproduction which were taboo. Such attitudes also made male access to childbirth more difficult. As Versluysen (1981: 29) argues, 'the gross indecency, violation of female modesty and the very threat to married life supposedly occasioned by male access to the female body during labour and delivery was frequently raised by critics of male-midwives'.

Male-midwives thus challenged established sexual mores concerning body contact. The paradigm of medical knowledge of the time furthermore, stressed reporting of symptoms by the patient rather than clinical examination (Foucault, 1973). The market which male-midwives were aiming to capture was the fee-paying middle and upper class patients. In such an interaction 'patronage' was likely to be the basis for practitioner-patient interaction (Johnson, 1972). Most patients were likely to be of similar or superior status and thus the man-midwife had little control over client preferences. For all these reasons male control over parturition was not easily established and specific strategies were developed to overcome them. A major strategy mentioned was the creation of lying-in hospitals by men-midwives. These charitable institutions received only patients of lower status than the male-midwives themselves. With an assured supply of clinical material, the male-midwife was able to press his claim for greater recognition amongst his medical colleagues and greater use of his services in the fee-paying (ie middle and upper class) part of the obstetric market (Verslysen, 1981).

Thus the overall process of a transition in the attendance of childbirth from untrained working class women to formally trained petit-bourgeois men was begun before the settlement of Australia commenced. The position of midwifery as a lower status health occupation was also fixed before settlement began. It is important to note also that the basic features of the relationship between medicine and midwifery had evolved before the advances in the understanding of childbirth which came to be known as part of 'scientific medicine'.

As Oakley (1976: 38) comments, 'the alliance of surgery with male-midwifery and the exclusion of women from formal medical and surgical training formed the basis on which female-midwifery was recognised as a secondary status health profession'.

Most accounts of this early period stress a form of technological determinism to explain this period of transition. The public appearance of forceps it is argued, (eg Radcliffe, 1967: 56) was crucial in the medical conquest of midwifery and came to symbolise the art of the obstetrician. As elsewhere, I would oppose this explanation. As Versluysen (1981: 30) argues,

> Since historians of midwifery have generally been obstetricians it is hardly suprising that they would stress the technical progress represented by the forceps. However it is hardly likely that a single isolated advance could have accounted for the medical conquest of midwifery.

As evidence she cites the practices of a number of men-midwives of the period to show that forceps were little utilised. Dr Smellie for instance, a major figure amongst male-midwives of the period and the person responsible for popularising the use of forceps, claimed to have used them in only ten cases out of 10 000 deliveries. She concludes:

> although the obstetric forceps would have given medical men the advantage in a few complicated or laborious deliveries, in general the abuse of midwifery instruments including the forceps by less skilled doctors, discredited medical midwives as a whole exposing them to criticism and hostility from many quarters, and is one of the main themes of the opponents of medical midwifery. (Versluysen, 1981: 31)

Rather than determining the medical conquest of midwifery, the popularisation of forceps by male practitioners was one of the strategies adopted in the struggle with midwives. The potential availability of forceps should complications arise, could be stressed as the major reason why male-midwives should be employed.

The pioneer era to 1880

In the case of doctors there is a considerable amount of information on who migrated to Australia, but the same is not true of midwives. There is little information on how many trained, or untrained but experienced midwives made the journey. In her study of midwives in the United States, Kobrin (1966) argues that few midwives emigrated there. As Australia was often second choice after the United States for emigrants from the United Kingdom, it seems reasonable to assume that even fewer migrated to Australia.

There were no midwives recorded as having been among the 191 female convicts on the First Fleet in 1788 which marks the beginning of white settlement of Australia. The census of 1814 however does mention one Phoebe Norton as being a midwife in Parramatta. Phoebe Norton was 26-years-old when transported with her son for stealing spoons and bed linen to the value of 31 shillings while in service.

In an attempt to segregate the sexes, the Female Factories were built at Parramatta outside Sydney and at Cascade near Hobart. Forster (1967: 11) argues that these must be recognised as Australia's first maternity institutions, as convict women went there to be confined. The pregnancy rate among female convicts he argues, was high and the staff included a permanent midwife who was known in the convict flash-slang as a 'fingersmith'. Undoubtedly a number of convict women became midwives out of necessity. There is a report of one such part-time midwife convict, Margaret Catchpole, who was in domestic service initially but later involved in 'farming, nursing and helping settlers' wives bring their babies into the light of the colonial sun' (Pownall, 1964: 44).

An early example of conflict between a midwife and a doctor, and one that was often to be repeated was recorded in 1804 at Parramatta. A midwife attending a settler, sent for a surgeon, John Savage, to attend because of a difficult labour requiring forceps and skilled assistance. Savage refused to attend, claiming there were no forceps available, and rode off to Sydney. The woman subsequently died and Savage was court-martialled for neglect of duty, found guilty, dismissed from service and sent back to England, though the sentence was later set aside as it was contended the offence was not in a strict sense a military one (Forster, 1967: 13). As Forster indicates, cases of refusal by doctors to come to cases where midwives were in attendance were reported from elsewhere also, though it is likely that as well as an anti-midwife element, such an incident may also have reflected the arrogance and neglect which was a feature of class relations of the time.

Settlement soon spread from Sydney as settlers pushed inland and south in search of good grazing lands. The conditions of childbirth for these early rural pioneers were very difficult. Often there was no skilled assistance of either doctor or midwife available at all and women had to make do with help from their husbands or each other. Indeed there are numerous accounts of Aboriginal women acting as midwives for settler women in childbirth. This very early sisterhood among Australian women with assistance at childbirth would appear to be one of the few examples of assistance being provided across both class and colour lines. Pownall (1964), in her account of pioneer women argues that 'stories of native women who acted as emergency midwives appear in every district'.

Other pioneer women 'neighboured' each other as a number of diaries and letters which have survived show. Letters from an early pioneer woman in the Parramatta district, Harriet King, to her husband demonstrate this:

> May 1828: I have been in Paramatta lately attending dear Mary [her sister-in-law]; who has been a sufferer indeed. I staid with her a month, then went home for a fortnight, went in again, staid a week, came home and was sent for again as she was confined to her bed ... Nov. 1828: Mary is again en famille and expects to be confined about April or May, I am to be in attendance.
>
> (Teale, 1978: 71)

Childbirth must have been a considerable ordeal for pioneer women especially as doctors in country areas were few and far between and experienced midwives more so. On the other hand, even when some medical care became available, it was often not used as Ada Cambridge (1903: 104) has argued:

> Speaking of those Bush babies, I would point out that medical attendance was in the category of non essential luxuries that are now necessaries of life in very class. When it cost a little fortune and the waste of days to get a doctor, the struggling Bushman's wife, as a rule took her chance without him. Occasionally she was conveyed to the nearest township which possessed one and there awaited in lodgings the opportunity to profit by his services; but the majority of Bush women preferred to stay at home and make shift with the peripatetic Gamp [sic] old and unscientific as she always was.

Mention should be made here of the literary stereotype referred to on this occasion; that of Sairey Gamp a character from a Dickens novel. Of his character Dickens wrote (in 1871):

> The face of Mrs Gamp—the nose in particular—was somewhat red and swollen and it was difficult to enjoy her society without becoming conscious of a smell of spirits. Like most persons who have obtained a great eminence in their profession, she took to hers very kindly, insomuch that, setting aside her natural predilections as a woman, she went to a lying-in or a laying-out with equal zest and relish.

This stereotype was widely used by opponents of independent midwifery to describe midwives in general (at times), but particularly 'untrained' ones. Its usage must be seen as an attempt to discredit midwives as a whole and as an element in the strategy of male medical takeover.

The argument has been made by Forster (1967) that the care of women in labour has always been largely in the hands of doctors, in contrast to the situation in Europe. This claim has been picked up and reproduced uncritically by others such as Teale (1978). However neither provide any evidence to support their contention and certainly it would not on the face of it apply either to rural areas, where there were few doctors available, or to working class urban areas where the doctor's fee was difficult if not impossible to manage.

The process that occurred especially in rural areas and indeed was exemplified in the Omeo and Mansfield districts was that on initial settlement women mainly assisted each other and 'freely gave help during sickness and childbirth' (Prendergast, 1968: 41). As the local community developed, one or two women began to specialise, based on having had children themselves and having assisted at the birth of many others. This 'wise woman' type of midwife sometimes took up midwifery as a means of supporting herself following the death of a spouse. Payment was sometimes made in money, more often in kind, and sometimes not at all. One such midwife documented by Gillison (1974), in her account of the Mansfield area, was Elizabeth Noar of Gaffney's Creek who came from Manchester in 1849 with her husband and two sons. Her husband died in Melbourne and she journeyed to the Gaffney's Creek goldfield in 1862 with her son and daughter-in-law. She soon gained a reputation as a skilled midwife and was much sought after in the area.

The third stage in the development of midwifery services occurred when a doctor arrived in the area and a more formal medical division of labour emerged. Usually this involved the midwife attending most confinements, with the doctor available if complications arose or an instrument delivery (ie forceps) was indicated. The doctor also usually attended the confinements of the more affluent in the town. Only the squatter's wife would on occasion travel out of the district to the regional centre or to Melbourne to be delievered. In the urban areas by contrast different conditions prevailed on account of the greater availability of doctors. Midwives mainly attended the confinements of working class women who could not afford to pay the doctor's fee which in 1877 was recommended as a minimum of three guineas (AMJ, 1877: 132). In 1880 the wage of labourers was only six to seven shillings per day (Victorian Year Book, 1883–1884).

The conflict over the appropriate occupational division of labour in attendance at childbirth between midwives and doctors in this early period of settlement, was related to the doctors' attempts to professionalise as a means of gaining upward social mobility. In their opposition to the practice of midwifery by midwives it is undoubtedly the case that an important component of the doctors' motivation in attempting to control midwives resulted from their perceived concern for maternal and infant welfare. No one would deny that midwives, being 'untrained', on occasion were responsible for unnecessary mortality amongst mothers and children, or indeed that on occasions there were flagrant cases of ignorance of proper procedures and ghastly mistakes made.

However, another important component of their motivation was the fear of competition which the cheap and popular local midwife provided. Furthermore, the claim that midwives were ignorant and dangerous was used as an ideological weapon in the struggle for control over childbirth, even in the face of available evidence to the contrary. The concern of the medical profession also rang hollow in view of their continued failure to provide any systematic training of midwives. As Forster (1967: 15) argues, this was an important factor in the maintenance of the pre-eminence of doctors in the obstetrical area; '. . . there were heated arguments over what form training, if instituted should assume, because many doctors feared that the fully qualified midwife would not only take over obstetrical practice, but also invade the lucrative field of diseases of women'.

As we have seen previously, doctors faced competition in the childbirth area not only from midwives, but also from unqualified practitioners of other sorts. That these so-called 'quacks' were attending confinements is beyond doubt from the records of court cases where they faced manslaughter charges resulting from these attendances (see Bowden, 1974: 175). The attendance of midwives was opposed by doctors partially at least because of the precedent they set for other unqualified *men* to take up midwifery. 'If ignorant women are to be allowed to practise midwifery, ignorant men are pretty sure to claim the same privilege and if the privilege may be claimed by an man, it can hardly be withheld from pharmaceutical chemists' (AMJ, Dec., 1871: 373).

Thus chemists also became caught up in the struggle over whose appropriate occupational territory was childbirth. Midwifery became in fact the lowest status occupation seeking parturition as its occupational territory. Its practitioners were by definition women and in particular, working class women. Indeed midwives were frequently the scapegoats in other struggles. The example was related earlier of a new arrival being offered for sale the certificate of a recently deceased medical man and being assured that midwives would receive the blame in any 'bad lying-in case' (Kelly, 1859: 71).

Indeed this notion of legal responsibility is an interesting one. In 1864 there was a case reported of a midwife who was convicted for manslaughter in a midwifery case where the mother had died. In her evidence, she said she had sent for a surgeon when she realised the birth was going to be difficult, but he had refused to come because he was not guaranteed payment (AMJ, 1864: 350–351). *She* was nonetheless culpable.

In 1856 a lying-in hospital was opened in Melbourne based upon the English model, including male medical staff and the provision of clinical training for medical students. In 1862 training for midwives to operate under male medical control was established. As in England where the model originated, the 'ladies' monthly nurse' who was the result of this training was more of a maternity nurse than a midwife. Forster (1967: 15) comments that the training was only a half measure because of this: 'The ladies' monthly nurse was a phenomenon of the Victorian era, an age when respectable childbirth always occurred at home because it was the safest place.' She was called a monthly nurse because that was how long she stayed, being involved more with the care of the mother and the running of the household than with the actual confinement which was attended by the doctor. She was thus subordinated to the doctor from the start and was not trained to act independently. Of course only the wealthy could afford her services and thus her impact was fairly limited. Some nurses trained in this way did take up practice as midwives however, contrary to the intentions of the doctors running the training course. This led to an angry editorial in the *Australian Medical Journal* (1877: 304): 'Some of these nurses so trained as monthly nurses have adopted the calling of midwives, using the certificates given to them as evidence of their right and competency to do so.'

The Medical Registration Act of 1862 was the first regulation which allowed 'qualified' medical practitioners to be differentiated from 'unqualified ones'. The grandfather clause however allowed entry into the medical profession for some who, though not formally trained had been in practice a number of years in Victoria prior to 1862. Any male-midwives there were, would seem to have been able to qualify on this basis (though none could be found), whereas female-midwives could not. Professionalisation of medicine at this stage then was accompanied by its genderisation.

There appears to have been considerable public support for midwives however, as exemplified by the Byaduk case near Belfast (now Port Fairy) in 1872. A local woman Margaret Thomson, had engaged the elderly district midwife Charlotte Ward (who had 30 years experience) at her confinement 'to save the doctor's bill'. Complications occurred which resulted in the local doctor being called in to assist, to no avail as it turned out as both the mother and child died. On the doctor's evidence, Mrs Ward was tried for manslaughter for alleged errors in her treatment. The medical facts of the case are unclear, even today as Forster (1965) shows. The point is however that the defence made an appeal to popular sentiment, stressing that Mrs Ward was well-known and much respected in the local district and hinted at victimisation, which, Forster suggests, helped the jury to return a popular verdict of 'not guilty'. The local newspaper, the *Belfast Gazette*, commented of the case:

> The public, while of course unable to obtain any reply will yet naturally ask why Mrs Ward an aged nurse and midwife, of much experience and irreproachable character, should be dragged before a jury and judge, compelled to undergo much mental anxiety and incur great expense and to suffer loss through withdrawal of patronage ... The only reasonable inference to be drawn is that the poor woman belongs to a class which is not in favour with doctors, more especially those who have but limited experience with midwifery. (Quoted in Forster, 1965: 1052)

By the end of the period under present consideration opposition to midwives from some sections of the medical profession was hardening. An editorial in the *Australian Medical Journal* in 1879 revealed medical opposition to any form of regulation and registration of midwives, also questioning 'whether the practice of obstetrics should be permitted to women at all' (AMJ, June, 1879: 285–287). In fact medical opposition was to prevent any form of registration for midwives until 1915. Unlike the English context however, where training in midwifery was not a required part of medical training until 1886, in Victoria it was from the start. When the Melbourne Medical School began in 1862, midwifery was part of the curriculum from the outset, though there was frequent criticism of the training provided. The different conditions in Australia, the lack of an established medical elite who opposed midwifery training and the necessity for Victorian doctors to engage in midwifery because of a shortage of trained attendants, would appear to explain this difference. The effect was that the general practitioner very quickly emerged as a competitor for the midwife.

The transition era 1880–1910

This period is marked by the evolution of nursing as an occupation and its attempts to incorporate midwifery within it. Associated with this was the expansion of training of midwives and the beginning of the registration issue which was to develop in the next era. These developments took place however, against a backdrop in which many of the features of the previous period remain important. Although no definitive figures are available, Pensabene (1980) suggests they would have attended well over half of all confinements. By this time specialisation had often occurred to the point where some local women became known as midwives and were able to earn a living from attending at confinements. It was also the period which saw in effect the beginning of the 'private maternity hospitals' where the local midwife began to use part of her own residence to deliver babies, rather than attending women in their own homes. Often this was advertised as well, with newspaper advertising beginning to appear in the 1880s of the sort: 'Accouchments—Mrs Moir is prepared to accommodate ladies at her residence, Pedrotta Terrace' (Thornton, 1972: 22).

Amongst doctors too, obstetrics continued to be regarded as a low status branch of medicine. 'There still remains something of a tendency to look upon midwifery as a branch of practice which any man can take on without fear of failure' (Jamieson, 1885: 206). This appears to have been reflected in the teaching of midwifery to medical students. Although the Melbourne Medical School was quite advanced in requiring training in midwifery from the outset in 1862, the extent to which this actually ensured proficiency among new medical graduates was questionable. An Australian surgeon, recalling his medical training in obstetrics in the late nineteenth century reveals this:

Since our practical work was limited to a dozen actual midwifery cases, we graduated after passing an examination in theoretical obstetrics, without really knowing how to confine a woman. Every one of us, after qualification went to his first midwifery case, trying to comfort himself with the thought that 90 per cent of deliveries came head first. We also secretly resolved to be *fussily inactive* while the old midwife helped the woman through. At least we could always contrive to look wise. (Moran, 1939: 92; emphasis added)

In line with the development of 'scientific medicine' in general, the advances made in the understanding of disease filtered through to the obstetrical area and led to changes in the medical curriculum, though as in other areas there was a considerable time lapse between the discovery and introduction of new methods of treatment and their widespread usage. Changes were made to the medical curriculum during this time which reflected the changing understanding of midwifery, and the gradual acceptance of parturition as an appropriate, indeed important part of the occupational territory of medicine. More emphasis gradually came to be placed on clinical experience and training (Forster, 1967: 35; Russell, 1977: 90).

Alongside developments in the training of medical students in obstetrics, the training of midwives also developed during the 1880s, becoming more formalised. The male medical staff provided formal instruction in midwifery although their intention was the creation not of an independent midwife, but a subordinated maternity nurse. The type of health worker intended at the time as actually akin to the modern midwife, with general basic nursing training followed by specialised instruction in midwifery.

Certainly however some midwives who were in practice availed themselves of the opportunity to undertake formal instruction in midwifery. Mary Howlett was one such midwife in the Lake Bolac district, 160 miles west of Melbourne. Mary Howlett had taken up midwifery in 1866 on the urging of the local doctor and had practised for over 50 years. In 1887, she undertook the six month training course at the age of 46 years. As Forster (1965: 1050) recounts,

> Mrs Howlett returned to her home near Lake Bolac and practised in this district as a nurse and midwife ... she attended up to ten or twelve cases per annum and her usual fee was three guineas but she often was not fully paid. She went to her patient at the onset of labour and stipulated that she should be called for with a horse and buggy ... In her earlier years of practice she would stay for about nine days after delivery and the mother was kept strictly in bed for this time; but later she usually remained three days.

In 1888 however as a result of pressure from the government, public opinion and some sections of the medical profession, the system of training was changed and the first course specifically in midwifery was begun at the Women's Hospital. The medical staff however were opposed to the training of independent midwives. The Diploma in Midwifery which was established in 1893 could be taken only after general nurse training. This enabled the medical staff to keep close control over the practice of midwives. Through the 1880s and 1890s midwifery training was increasingly incorporated with nursing. In 1898 the title obstetrical nurse replaced 'ladies' monthly nurse'. In 1899 it was decided that only those who had taken general nursing training would be employed in the hospital's midwifery department. Both doctors and nurses agreed on this it is important to note; nurses because it extended their occupational territory to include the tasks associated with childbirth, doctors because the incorporation of midwifery into nursing ensured its subordination.

Not only in training was the incorporation of midwifery occurring, but also in practice as well. In 1885 the Melbourne District Nursing Service had been set up along the charitable lines common at the time to provide medical service for the 'deserving' (ie not unmarried mothers) sick poor (see Rosenthal, 1974). The 1890s depression convinced the society of the need to set up a home midwifery service for those unable to avail themselves of the facilities provided in the Women's Hospital or to afford attendance by doctors. This was explicitly done to take midwifery out of the hands of the untrained midwife. A charge of £1 was made and a midwifery nurse attended when summoned and gave all medical attention for two to three weeks after the birth. A roster of doctors was organised to provide back up support if required.

Further developments in the relationship between midwifery and nursing took place in the early years of the twentieth century. The first occupational association of nurses was set up in 1901—the Victorian Trained Nurses Association (VTNA), joining organisations in other states in 1902 to form the Australian Trained Nurses Association (ATNA) (Centenary of Nurse Training in Victoria, 1962). The nurses followed the model of professionalisation provided by the doctors in an attempt to gain upward social mobility for its members. Their strategy followed that of the doctors in setting up a register, beginning publication of their own journal (*Una*), advocating standards of training and seeking legal support through a registration act. The questions of the relationship between nurses and doctors was one which was well settled by this time. The subordination of nursing stemmed from the days of Florence Nightingale. In her initial nursing exercise in the Crimean war, Nightingale from the outset refused to attend patients unless directed by doctors. Nursing thus came into being as a subordinate occupation and largely has remained that way since.

The passing of a Midwives Registration Act in 1902 in the United Kingdom provided considerable stimulation to the debate. The VTNA came out strongly against such an act in Victoria, as the effect would be to create an occupation of midwifery, separate and independent to nursing. An article in *Una* (the nurses' journal) claimed that the number of untrained women practising midwifery in Victoria was small (though no evidence was presented) and argued that the need for midwives could best be met by an outdoor maternity service from the Women's Hospital, such as the District Nursing Service. The article also defended the training of obstetric nurses rather than midwives at the hospital (quoted in Centenary of Nurse Training in Victoria, 1962: 22). The claim that few untrained midwives were in practice does not however appear to be supported by the evidence. Indeed in 1904, the head of the medical staff at the hospital could claim that 'We find that a very large section of the community chiefly for financial reasons, is given over to the care of those untrained women, who are classed, not inappropriately as "Sairey Gamps" ' (quoted in Centenary of Nurse Training in Victoria, 1962: 25). The lady superintendent in the same year wrote: 'Something must eventually be done to stem the flood of Gampians, and the sooner we face the situation and its difficulties the better. The Gamp is not dying out, for every day of my experience brings fresh proof of the numbers that are entering into the running.' (quoted in Centenary of Nurse Training in Victoria, 1962: 26)

The question of the training of midwives thus represented a considerable problem for nursing as it emerged. Trained midwifery nurses could not be trained quickly enough to satisfy the demand for midwifery services and the Women's Hospital was under considerable pressure, again from the state government, to lower its standard of training so that practising midwives could be given some training in midwifery. Both nursing and medicine opposed this, because it would be likely to lead to an independent occupation outside the control of doctors and competing with it. The occupational territory of such an independent occupation would overlap with that of both medicine and the emerging nursing occupation.

As well as this conflict with nursing, the conflict between medicine and midwifery also continued through this period. In January 1894, there was a report of a court case in Prahran where a local doctor on behalf of the Victorian Branch of the BMA prosecuted a midwife in the area, Lydia Littlefield, for unqualified medical practice. The case was dismissed however after the defence claimed that a midwife was not a medical practitioner and did not come within the classification of medical titles requiring registration. An editorial in the *Australian Medical Gazette* (15.7.1894: 241–242) criticised the doctor for bringing such a 'hopeless' case, calling the prosecution 'paltry'. The article called for the registration of midwives in Australia, supporting their right to practise. 'There are thousands of poor women in these colonies who cannot afford to pay for a medical man's attendance, but who could manage to give a midwife something to secure their services for a small time which is a woman's hour of greatest need, to whom the existence of midwives is a Godsend.'

Some medical practitioners undoubtedly did support the midwife and her continued existence and called for her better education. A Townsville doctor in 1891 for example, showing that 73 per cent of all births in the Townsville district in 1890 were attended by midwives alone, argued 'this proves there is a demand for midwives and would be impossible to attempt to do away with them. We cannot compel a woman to have a doctor, therefore we must put up with them' (Nisbet, 1891: 270–271). He went on to call for their education and registration, education into a definite place in the division of labour:

> An ideal nurse or midwife would be one whose powers of diagnosis of normal and abnormal conditions were fully trained and founded on long experience, but whose knowledge of treatment outside a normal case was nil, so that she might never be tempted to venture on ground belonging to the skilled obstetrician, and requiring an intimate knowledge of the principles of medicine and surgery.

Yet while there was a section of the medical profession that supported the independent status of the occupation of midwifery within health care, this would appear to have been a small minority, and most clearly did not. When the idea of registration for midwives was mooted in 1908 *The Intercolonial Medical Journal* (20.11.1909: 572–573) invited comment from readers, estimating that 37 per cent of all births were attended by midwives. The invitation drew sharp response in the next issue, in a letter signed 'Self Preservation'.

> I have a practice the 'backbone' of which is undoubtedly midwifery. I am against a class of women being registered as above, because I learnt when on a recent visit to England that this branch of work is fast slipping away from the medical man. The public get the idea the midwife's training and skill is exactly the same as the doctor, and, seeking a saving in money, they naturally engage only a midwife. The doctor is called in when the eleventh hour strikes—called in Sir, to save the midwife at her suggestion. Often these eleventh hour operations are extremely risky as regards the patient; the case does badly and the medical profession gets another pushdown.
>
> (IMJA, 20.1.1909: 631–633)

The doctor in question preferred untrained midwives as they were less of a competitor saying 'very soon a medico gets the ordinary midwife into clean habits. Anyway I have a splendid record and not one of my nurses has been "trained" or "examined"'.

In the development of Australian capitalism, the turn of the century marks the growing involvement by the state in a number of areas of the economy, including the health system, which had previously been left largely to the operation of market forces. A concern with the quantity and condition of labour power became apparent, and through the early part of the twentieth century there were numerous royal commissions and commissions of inquiry which investigated the condition and development of the Australian population. The evolution of the 'populate or perish' ethos led to a concern with the declining birth rate in Australia (see Hicks, 1978). The 1904 Royal Commission on the 'Decline of the Birth Rate and Mortality of Infants in New South Wales' was the first of many such investigations. Maternal and child welfare became a matter of national importance and action was encouraged on these grounds rather than just humanitarian ones. The midwife was blamed by the commission as having been responsible for much of the maternal and infant mortality. With strong biblical overtones she was defined as being 'surgically unclean' almost by definition and the practice of midwifery, it was recommended, should be restricted to medical practitioners and 'trained midwifery nurses, who should be subject to examination, licence and medical control' (NSW PP, 1, 1904: 32; see also Pringle, 1973: 19–27).

Elsewhere however, and when it came to actually framing legislation to regulate health occupations, the inability of medical practitioners to actually take medical control in all cases especially in rural areas, as well as the laissez-fair notion that women should be able to choose whoever they wanted to attend them in childbirth, operated to prevent a medical monopoly of attendance at childbirth being attained. The 1908 Medical Registration Act in Victoria exemplifies this. The deputation from the BMA which met with the Chief Secretary Sir Samuel Gillott to lobby for the act, wanted as part of that act a ban on all 'unqualified' practice. This was strongly opposed by the Chief Secretary who argued on one hand that it was a precedent which existed nowhere else and ran against the principles on which other acts had been based. On the other hand he argued, such a ban would affect midwives, who he considered were of crucial importance to the state. 'There are parts of the state where there is no medical man within miles and women have to do this work.' (CSO, 05/V6560, 15.11.1905) Midwives were thus not affected by the act, despite the opposition of the medical profession. Although the 1908 act was important in giving the medical profession dominance within the health system, the role of midwives as reproducers of labour power particularly in rural areas, prevented their being excluded altogether. This was despite the wishes of the medical profession.

The greatest single cause of maternal deaths throughout the nineteenth century and into the twentieth century was puerperal fever, a type of septic poisoning which began in the uterus and was created by the separation of the placenta. The precautions necessary to prevent this dreaded disease were actually discovered in the late eighteenth century but it was not until the work of Semmelweis and Lister had filtered through into medical practice that it was fully understood. Such a filtering through was retarded by the obstinacy of the medical profession in not adopting the simple precautions of washing their hands and changing their clothes after each delivery. Semmelweis, as is well known, was ridiculed for suggesting (based on a controlled trial) that doctors might be responsible for persistence of puerperal fever. Yet half a century later in 1906, the medical training received by students at Sydney University (at least) was devoid of any appreciation of the work of Semmelweis (Moran, 1939). Epidemics of puerperal fever occurred throughout the nineteenth century and into the twentieth century and many public hospitals refused to take maternity patients because of the fear of this dreaded disease. The midwife became an easy scapegoat to blame for the outbreaks of puerperal fever, as was the case with the findings of the New South Wales 1904 Royal Commission. In fact however the more affluent middle class women attended by doctors ran a greater risk of infection than did the poorer women attended by the midwife.

In the specialised maternity hospitals such as the 'Women's', stringent precautions were taken to attempt to prevent the incidence of infection. Before 1875 for example, there was a rigid distinction made between infirmary and midwifery nurses. There was no interchange of personnel on a day-to-day basis; they even ate in different dining rooms. While nurses were rigidly divided as early as 1875 however, the same precautions were not thought to be necessary for doctors, and for a further thirteen years until 1888, doctors could move freely between the infirmary and midwifery sections of the hospital; an historical example of the argument made in the medical sociology literature by Julius Roth (1957). Roth's observation was that the higher status the personnel involved, the less contagious they are thought to be—that is, the most stringent contagion controls are required of the lowest status participants and vice versa. Yet throughout this period claims continued that puerperal fever was the result of the practice of midwives, a claim that was used to justify the call for the exclusion of midwives from attending childbirth. The ideological nature of this claim was revealed in the next period when there was widespread recognition that the midwife was less to blame than had been assumed.

The takeover period

The final period to be analysed is from 1910 till the late 1930s, the period when doctor domination of midwifery was extended and achieved in a more complete fashion than previously. The 'reproduction', it will be argued, came about in considerable part as a result of a greater state concern for maternal and infant welfare which led to state patronage for the medical profession as they consolidated themselves into a position of dominance and control over other occupations within the health systems. The subordination of midwifery was formally achieved by its 'limitation' in various midwifery registration acts from 1915 to 1920, and its final and formal incorporation into nursing in 1928.

The growing state concern with the health of its labour force was reflected in a number of Western countries in the payment of a maternity allowance to mothers for each child produced. This 'baby bonus' as it was known, was designed both to encourage parents to have more children and also to provide a sum of money so that assistance at childbirth could be afforded by all. The passing of the 'Maternity Allowance Act' in Australia in 1912 is of major interest to us here because of the influence it executed on the social organisation of childbirth. The Commonwealth Parliamentary debates over the introduction of the bill demonstrate the government's growing concern with the welfare of its citizens. It also marks the beginnings of state responsibility for health which was a feature of the transition from laissez-faire to monopoly capitalism.

The need to increase the birth rate and thereby the population was seen as necessary to avoid the 'race suicide' which was thought to be looming. The 'baby bonus' thus represented an incentive to couples to have larger families. The then Attorney-General and future Prime Minister, Billy Hughes, argued 'The bill is a recognition of the value of children to the state and the services rendered by mothers in producing them' (CPD, 66, 1911: 3338). He went on to justify the growth of state interventions in the health area, saying:

> It is the business of the state to look after its people and it is a short sighted and wholly wrong system of economics that teaches that the best results flow from allowing the individual to do as best he can without guidance and without aid. We see clearly enough these days when production had developed so tremendously that the state must interfere in certain directions. (CPD, 66, 1911: 3339)

That the intention of the act was primarily economic and not humanitarian is revealed by the fact that the allowance (a 'fiver') was not payable to Aboriginal or Asiatic women living in Australia, nor to Papuan women in Australia's colony. Also the notion of a 'viable' child was introduced. The payment was not made in the case of a child which was stillborn or lived less than twelve hours.

The medical profession came out in opposition to the bonus. An editorial in the *Medical Journal of Australia* (13.2.1915: 151) claimed that a 'fiver' was too lavish and its payment should be means tested. It also claimed that it was likely to lead to an increase in the patronage of midwives.

> By giving to practically every lying-in woman the sum of five pounds, a large amount of money is made available for attendance on women during this period. The medical practitioner is proverbially a bad businessman, but the half trained or wholly untrained midwife is as keen as any shark in the cities. These women are attracted by the prospect of picking up a substantial portion of the 'fiver' and consequently lure prospective mothers to engage their services, either in their own homes or at the 'house' of the so called midwife.

The consequences, the editorial argued, would be an increase in puerperal fever: 'The incidence of sepsis will undoubtedly increase in proportion to the increase of untrained or half trained midwives who "assist" the women in childbirth.' On both counts however the result of the introduction of the baby bonus was the exact opposite of what the doctors believed. The proportion of births attended by midwives, decreased, and the incidence of puerperal fever was scarcely altered. The introduction of the maternity allowance made exact figures on birth attendance calculable for the first time from its returns (Barrett,

1923: 121–126). The proportion of births attended solely by midwives was halved in the decade following, both in Victoria and also in the Commonwealth as a whole. The £5 handout removed the financial barrier to medical attendance and a greater proportion of women preferred to have a doctor confine them than a midwife. However, this did not lead to a marked reduction in the maternal and infant mortality rate. The introduction of the baby bonus in 1913 also led to no substantial decrease in the puerperal death rate. Approximately one woman in 200 died just after its introduction and the same number a decade later. The case is similar with infantile mortality, where again there was only a small reduction. Thus while the proportion of births attended by doctors increased considerably, the maternal and infant mortality rates were scarcely affected.

Recognition of the falsity of linking midwives with puerperal fever was slow in coming however. Noting that by 1916 the maternity allowances were costing the Commonwealth upwards of three quarters of a million pounds each year, a Commonwealth committee of inquiry into maternal mortality recommended that the money would be better spent strengthening medical control over the childbirth process—that is the 'provision of trained attention by properly qualified and *properly supervised* midwife or nurse during the lying-in period' (CPP, 1917: 1014; emphasis added). Other suggestions for improving the 'productivity' of the baby bonus, which also had the effect of strengthening medical control included making it payable only if the woman consulted a doctor, and using the money to set up prematernity clinics over which doctors had control (see Thame, 1974).

The 'takeover' of the midwifery area was thus influenced by factors outside the health system itself; factors more related to reproduction and legitimacy concerns at the level of the state, particularly in rural areas. A similar argument can be made with regard to the registration of midwives in 1915 which temporarily gave the occupation an independent status, and to the 1928 Registration Act which saw the formal incorporation of midwifery into nursing.

The Midwives Registration Bill was introduced into the Victorian Parliament in early 1915, following agreement between the Australian Trained nurses Association (ATNA) and the management committee of 'The Womens' (Armstrong 1951: 186–215). The debate over the bill showed considerable confusion over the occupational boundary with nurses, and the difference between obstetrical nurses and midwives (VPD, 140, 1915: 1860). The confusion was exacerbated by the fact that a bill to register nurses was before the parliament at the same time. The nurses were unsuccessful at this time however, it appears because of the need for midwives in rural areas.

The Midwives Act passed in 1915 thus came about not so much as a result of pressure from midwives themselves but through support from other sources. The government negotiated the specific details of the bill with interested parties, amongst whom the medical management of the Women's Hospital appears to have been of most importance. At this time nursing was unsuccessful at claiming midwifery as its own occupational territory or indeed achieving registration itself. The state thus supported midwifery legislation over the ambitions of nursing.

The 1915 Act 'to provide for the Registration and Better Training of Midwives and to Regulate their Practice' placed considerable restrictions on the practice of midwives and brought them much more under medical control. Following the lines of the English act, a midwives board was appointed to make regulations governing the practice of midwifery. The Act provided for the registration of midwives with the intention of preventing unregistered persons calling themselves midwives, or attending childbirth for gain. Midwives had to be women, at least 23 years of age and able to satisfy the board they were of good character. Two grounds for registration were provided; either holding a qualification in midwifery or having been in 'bona fide' practice as a midwife for more than two years prior to the Act. This latter 'grandmother' clause which was also provided in the early registration acts of doctors, allowed the large number of 'untrained' midwives to achieve registration and thus continue in practice. On the first register, published in 1917, 83 per cent of the 700 names had qualified under this 'grandmother clause' (VGG, 2.2.1917: 520–528).

Considerable disciplinary powers were vested in the board. A midwife could be suspended if the board considered her a likely cause of the spread of infection (though compensation could be paid) and if the regulations about calling in a general practitioner were not followed. The Act carefully defined the occupational territory of midwifery as not to include the writing of medical or death certificates and 'cases of abnormality or disease in connection with parturition'. This latter limitation is significant as a form of deskilling, as it protected the doctors' monopoly as a social control agency.

Some of the requirements of the Act are important also in confirming the subordination of midwives vis-a-vis doctors. It was not required of doctors that they be of good character, and while they had to notify change of address, no time period was specified for this. Midwives however were required to notify change of address within three days, and furthermore, were required to pay an annual registration fee of five shillings, merely for the right to practise. No such fee was required of doctors in order to follow their occupation. Midwives, unlike doctors, were also not given the right to sue for non-payment of their fees. The 'regulations' the Act called for were published in the *Government Gazette* in June 1916. These are wideranging and covered the training of midwives and the conditions of practice. A curriculum of training over twelve months was set out which included invalid cookery and some general nursing training, including lectures on 'the distinctions between doctor's work and that of the nurse' (VGG, 14.6.1916: 2225). Under the conditions of practice which were set down, there is further illustration of the supposed selectivity of contagiousness according to the status of the practitioner involved. The midwife was required to bathe regularly in disinfectant, including washing her hair with disinfectant. No such procedures were required of doctors in order to attend childbirth.

A number of modifications were made to the 1915 Act, mainly reflecting concern over the shortage of midwives in rural areas. Blame was laid at the door of the medical profession in Parliamentary debates. The failure of doctors to take on the training of midwives was alleged to result from the continuing competition between doctors and midwives. It was argued that

> it is mainly because midwives enter into competition with them. That sort of thing should not be tolerated. There are many midwives who have had the necessary training and are more capable in certain cases than the average doctor. The medical profession indeed is very jealous of the midwives profession. There are many women who could carry out all the duties required provided the necessary training was given them. (VPD, 1919: 1923)

In 1923 the nurses, after a long battle by the RVTNA, finally got their own Registration Act. This Act demarcated the occupational boundary between midwifery and nursing. Nurses were not allowed to attend childbirth for gain whether under the direction of a medical practitioner or not, unless they were also eligible for registration under the Midwives Act. Provision was made for nurses to be eligible for registration as midwives, but only in country areas and then under certain fairly stringent conditions.

The independence of midwifery however was shortlived. In 1928 a further Act was passed which had the effect of formally incorporating midwifery as a special branch within nursing. Expediency was the main reason claimed for introducing the bill, but there is no doubt it was sought and supported by both nurses and doctors. Dr Stanley Argyle, the government spokesman, and also a doctor, claimed 'it is an essay on the part of the government to improve the position of midwives by handing over the matter of their control to an expert body known as the Nurses Board, which already controls the education of nurses and should deal therefore with a subject which is really a special branch of nursing' (VPD, 177, 1928: 1753).

Under the Act the Midwives Board was abolished and the control over the occupation of midwifery was vested in the Nurses Registration Board. The 1929 bill is of particular importance as it marks the end of midwifery as an independent occupation within the health system. Henceforth midwives would be first and foremost nurses. Incorporating it within nursing had the effect of subordinating it to medicine much more formally than had previously occurred. Its incorporation and thereby subordination had the effect of defending and extending 'medical dominance' within health care. The main competitor to medicine within a major area of medical work (obstetrics) was thereby controlled.

In the period during which these legislative changes took place, the relationship between midwifery and medicine continued to evolve at the day-to-day level. The themes of competition and rural shortages which were important in early periods continued during this time. Many doctors were nervous about the effect which the Midwives Registration Act would have on their practices, as letters to their journals indicate (eg MJA, 6.11.1915: 456). Such letters indicate that the Act had failed to curb the practice of unregistered midwives. One letter, signed 'Country Practitioner', complained that an unregistered midwife in his town was operating a private maternity hospital and advertising as well (MJA, 26.12.1921). Yet other doctors were helping to ensure the continued existence of unregistered midwives by continuing to attend when requested. A letter in 1921 wanted the BMA to declare it to be unethical for a doctor to attend unless the midwife was duly qualified. This he claimed he did, but complained that others did not follow this principle (MJA, 19.2.1921: 166).

Throughout this period the theme of rural shortage is a constant one, and in rural communities which could not attract a doctor, the midwife was a person of considerable status. As a result the subordination of midwives was a more gradual process in rural areas. In the parliamentary debate over the introduction of the Midwives Act of 1919 one member reminisced:

> I remember being in a remote township on the Upper Murray some years ago with a friend, who raised his hat to a woman we were passing. He told me she was the midwife of the district and they had to be careful not to do anything to make her leave the place because if she left it would be necessary to travel 60 miles to get somebody to take her place. (VPD, 153, 1919: 1926)

Further evidence is contained in the biography of Dr David Browne who practised in the Cobden area in the 1920s. An untrained midwife attended local confinements until he arrived. Not long after his arrival he attempt to get local support to raise funds for a cottage maternity hospital but, as he relates,

> a few subscriptions came in, none very big and it soon became apparent the project was lagging. In due course another public

meeting was called and this time the reason for the lagging became evident. It was noticeable there were present many who had shown no interest in the project until this meeting. One wondered and soon found out. These people at the meeting belaboured two themes; one 'what about the poor midwife being done out of a living and she being an old resident working in the village before this young doctor was born.' (Browne, 1976: 50)

The local people thus objected to the planned takeover by the young doctor, however good his intentions. Similar evidence is provided in the history of the Koo-Wee-Rup district in Gippsland (Mickle, 1979: Pellissier, 1979). Elderly local residents remember Ida Osborn, the local midwife who delivered them and the only nurse in the local area, which was comprised mainly of swampland. The nearest doctor was in Dandenong, 30 kilometres away, until a doctor settled in the area in 1914. Ida Osborn was very highly regarded in the area and continued to practise midwifery until 1928 however, to the chagrin of the new doctor as another resident recalled: 'The doctor was very put out by the choice of many mothers to engage Mrs Osborn to assist them at home rather than be admitted to the new "Bush nursing" hospital.' (quoted in Pellissier, 1979: 6).

There is considerable evidence also that despite the various registration acts, untrained and unregistered midwives (known as 'rabbit-snatchers') continued to practise in the country. The midwife referred to by Browne would appear to be in this category. He recalls that 'the local midwife had her patients in her home, simply a small over-crowded brick house. Her qualifications were simply that she had borne ten children of her own now all grown up' (Browne, 1976: 35). An example of the relative costs is given for the Victorian country town of Colac in 1926, when the cost of delivery by a midwife was reported to be two and a half guineas as against four guineas by a doctor. The midwife's relative cheapness was accentuated by the fact that confinement by the doctor in the local private hospital cost an additional five guineas weekly. By this time it was estimated only 50 per cent of confinements took place in the home (Brown, 1926: 476).

In the urban areas however the midwife continued to be important, but mainly only in working class areas. Marshall Allan (1928: 672) calculated from 1926 birth certificates that in 'residential' suburbs over 90 per cent were attended by doctors, whereas in poorer 'industrial' suburbs (Richmond, Collingwood, Fitzroy, Port Melbourne) the proportion was lower at 58 per cent to 88 per cent. He also calculated interesting figures for Victoria from birth certificates, showing in fact that the proportion delivered by midwives in the urban area was slightly higher than in country areas for most of the period, but that the takeover of attendance in confinements was, by 1926, occurring faster in the country than the city. In the urban areas then, working class women—midwives continued to attend the confinements of other women of their class. The 1917 register of midwives recorded only eight residential addresses of midwives in the upper and upper-middle class suburbs of Toorak and Kew, but 73 residential addresses from the working class suburbs of Collingwood, Richmond, Carlton and Fitzroy.

Early residents of Collingwood confirm this, indicating that most confinements in the area during this period were attended by midwives (Collingwood History Committee, 1979: 21). The Royal District Nursing Service also continued to be important during this period, surviving an attempt by the Women's Hospital to begin its own 'extern' maternity department staffed mainly by medical students, and protests from the BMA about the cheapness with which the society was attending midwifery patients (Rosenthal, 1974). The depression of the 1930s again led to an increase in demand for the services of the district nurses and midwives. In her oral record of the depression Lowenstein (1978: 22) quotes one informant's recollection of the time: 'Dulcie was born in a back room in the boarding house there. I didn't get to the hospital ... you had the old midwife come in. She was as rough as bags. If you had any money you'd give her a couple of pounds, or, if not you'd pay it off.'

For the state as a whole, a survey of general practitioners conducting midwifery in 1925 asked what proportion of births in the area were attended solely by midwives. Of the 116 replies to this question, over 50 per cent said either none or less than five per cent, while only eleven per cent indicated more than 30 per cent were (MJA, 21.3.1925: 295–297). At the official level, however, the takeover strategy continued.

Throughout this period doctors were trying to encourage women to be confined by doctors rather than midwives, using the ideology of professionalism to justify this takeover. Editorials such as the one appearing in the *Medical Journal of Australia* in 1921 were common and outlined the grounds for the attempted takeover.

> As soon as the wise woman recognises she is pregnant she consults her obstetrician and is prepared to follow his directions throughout the long months of her grossesse ... This is the action of the wise woman. The French employ this phrase 'sage femme' for someone quite different. The midwife or sage femme is not competent to guide the pregnant woman at this stage. A thorough knowledge of physiology and pathology is needed and there must be preparedness to apply special measures in the event of a pathological condition being discovered. It may not be practicable at the present time to make provision for the delivery of every woman under the guidance of a trained medical practitioner. But it is within the grounds of

practical politics to enable every pregnant woman to undergo observation by a medical practitioner during the second half of pregnancy. (MJA, 26.11.1921: 488–489)

Others attempted more direct strategies against midwives. In 1926 all the doctors in the South Australian town of Renmark united to insist that all their maternity patients be confined in hospital, and introduced a system of means-related fees to induce patients away from private midwives (Thame, 1974). This sort of strategy does not seem to have been very common however. In the hospital context medical control was well established; it was only in private, domiciliary practice that the midwife represented cheaper competition. Encouraging hospital confinement then was a means of establishing medical control over childbirth. The medicalisation of childbirth, a major feature of which was the move away from home births to hospital births, was closely associated with and indeed a major factor in the takeover of the childbirth area by doctors.

As we have seen, this was a period of great concern with maternal and infant welfare, and many reports and articles appeared on the theme of how to reduce the mortality of mothers and babies in childbirth. In this context the medical model was promoted as a strategy to justify medical attendance. Childbirth, it was stressed by some writers, was a dangerous 'medical' event. 'The immense amount of invalidism resulting from childbirth is immeasurable' (Jacobs, 1926: 595). Indeed this writer called for the abolition of even the term 'midwifery', arguing that 'the term midwifery should be now completely and for all time abolished when reference is made to this ascientific subject. Midwifery surely means the practice of midwives and unfortunately for our profession it comes to be regarded in this light'.

Through the decade of the 1920s there was a gradual realisation of the importance of ante-natal care for mothers, and as evidence of the ineffectualness of the baby bonus mounted despite the growing usage of doctors, there were many calls for the introduction of prematernity clinics, financed by the use of the money spent at the time on the baby bonus (see Thame, 1974). How these were to be run was left in no doubt.

It has been stated that maternity is the most important and most profitable industry of the human race. The industry should be protected by the application of real hygienic principles. The only way this can be effected with certainty is by the establishment in every convenient district of well equipped pre-maternity clinics placed in the charge of competent obstetricians. (MJA, 26.11.1921: 489)

The ideology of professionalism, including the claim to the

legitimacy of science, was the justification for this control. 'It must be remembered that the medical profession alone can carry out the work and that *freedom from lay interference is essential* ... Obviously no one other than a medical practitioner can be trusted to conduct these examinations. No nurse can have sufficient knowledge.' (MJA, 9.10.1926: 489; emphasis added)

Despite the evidence to the contrary, the tendency was still to blame the midwife for the infant and maternal mortality. Advances in medical science it was claimed, made the attendance of midwives at childbirth 'both a tradition and an anachronism' (Jacobs, 1926: 627) which should be done away with, some advocated, arguing 'therefore let the midwife attain the efficiency and gracefully assume the title of an obstetric nurse in whom the community and the medical profession will possess a real asset and will be proud to acknowledge' (Jacobs, 1926: 643).

The period under consideration is thus marked by intense competition between doctors and midwives. In a prize-winning essay the NSW director of maternal mortality, Dr E Morris, commented on the state of relations between the two occupations:

> The function of the midwife is to be the attendant of the woman whose pregnancy and confinement are normal. Theoretically the midwife is not a rival of the medical practitioner; in actual fact she is, nonetheless frequently regarded as such. So long as normal midwifery is considered a legitimate sphere of the medical practitioner and one especially which produces a sensible if not an essential portion of his income, this rivalry will continue. Instead of cooperation and complementary action between the midwife and the doctor we are apt to obtain distrust if not antagonism on both sides. Instead of the doctor being regarded by the untrained midwife as a blessing and a friend, she too frequently regards him as a necessary evil. (Morris, 1925: 309)

Yet this scapegoating of the midwife was misplaced as Morris went on to show. The maternal and infant mortality rate did not decline despite growing medical attendance. Two factors were associated with this. One was the continued deficiencies in the obstetrical training of medical students and the other was the over-enthusiasm of doctors in the use of the new medical technology associated with childbirth.

The education of medical students in obstetrics continued to be criticised during this period. Indeed this was one of the major factors pointed to by the various reports on maternal and infant mortality during this period. Obstetrics continued to be described as the 'Cinderella' of medicine throughout the period and indeed into the 1940s (Croll, 1924: 673–676); Shaw, 1947: 285); although from the mid-1920s the medical profession made a serious attempt to upgrade the teaching of obstetrics to medical students and also to improve the obstetrical work of the ordinary general practitioner.

The other problem with medical attendance at childbirth resulted paradoxically from developments in scientific medicine in the obstetrical area. Both anaesthesia and forceps as we have seen previously had been in use for a number of years, though their use by midwives was prohibited. The growing medical attendance at childbirth was accompanied by a somewhat over-enthusiastic use of these procedures to shorten labour and reduce the likelihood of infection, resulting in a proliferation of birth injuries to both mothers and infants. This was undoubtedly a major factor in accounting for the failure of doctors to lower the mortality and morbidity during this period. One New South Wales doctor boasted as late as 1929 that he had used forceps in all 768 deliveries over the last ten years in his practice, in order, he announced, to prevent complications occurring (Keveston, 1929: 14–19). As the New South Wales director of maternal and infant mortality lamented in his 1927 report,

> A disinclination on the part of the medical man to expedite delivery is apt to be misinterpreted as inefficient midwifery by a patient and her friends. A practitioner is liable to enhance his reputation by the almost universal use of forceps ... so long as one competitor adopts this practice, all others must show an equal competence. (NSW PP, 1927: 38)

He went on to estimate that in up to 50 per cent of cases attended by doctors, forceps were used. A call for a return to more natural delivery and the policy of 'masterly inactivity' gradually emerged. A letter to the *Medical Journal of Australia* (15.11.1930: 232) from a New South Wales country practitioner in 1930 claimed that it was humiliating that the midwife should get better results than the doctor and called for 1930 to be declared a 'no forceps year'.

By the 1930s, with the takeover of attendance at birth by doctors largely achieved, there was growing recognition that the midwife was not as much to blame as had been claimed. Some members of the profession, particularly in the public health area, had been saying this since the mid-1920s, but 1930 marks the end of the intense competition between doctors and midwives. Indeed a government report commissioned in 1930 into maternal welfare and carried out by a senior English public health official, Dame Janet Campbell, recommended a greater role for midwives in that normal cases should be left to them. She suggested that 'the advantages of such a proposition lie in the great skill and experience in normal delivery which can be gained by the trained midwives who are able to concentrate on a special branch of work to an extent which no doctor is likely to do' (Campbell, 1929–1930: 1535). Midwives she claimed, were more tolerant, sympathetic and understanding in the childbirth process than the male dominated medical profession. She also criticised the training of medical students, arguing that 'the tendency has also been to regard the new born baby as a somewhat unimportant byproduct, scarcely worth the attention of a busy obstetrician' (Campbell, 1929–1930: 1536).

By the 1930s the transformation in control over childbirth had occurred. From being an independent occupation, midwifery was transformed into a specialised branch of nursing and thereby subordinated to medicine.

The process of subordination

In explaining the wresting of control of parturition by the medical profession from formerly independent midwives, it could be argued, following Donnison (1977), that a distinction is necessary between attendance and management of childbirth. While doctors now manage confinement in an overall sense and are usually in attendance for the delivery itself, this is more of a ritual involvement and it is still the female midwives who attend and supervise the confinement as has always been the case. Contrary to this I would argue that while conceding the actual work done by midwives is little changed, the fact of male medical control over the encounter is crucial. Whereas previously doctors came to control the encounter in 'abnormal' circumstances, the control (manifested particularly in the notion of overall legal responsibility) has passed from the female-midwives to the male doctors.

How is this process outlined above to be explained? The main type of argument is a technological determinist one, and as in previous chapters I would specifically argue against this. Advances in the technology associated with childbirth did not provide the conditions under which the process occurred. Indeed in the birth area new techniques such as forceps delivery at times may have slowed it, especially through overuse. Rather, the subordination of midwives was achieved prior to advances in the understanding of childbirth. The takeover was slowed in fact by factors outside the medical system itself and resulting more from the political economy of Australian society, particularly the growing state concern with the reproduction of labour power. The argument that doctors needed to assume control over childbirth because only they could provide skilled assistance, rings hollow in the face of the refusal of the medical profession to provide training for midwives equal to that provided in other countries such as the United Kingdom.

Technological determinist explanations focus on the technical division of labour. Rather, I have argued in this study, it is necessary to focus on the relations of production and the social division of labour. Two elements of this social division of labour are relevant here. One is the gender of the participants. The takeover can be seen as a process of male medical imperialism, so that the health division of labour came to replicate the sexual division of labour in the domestic context with the male-husband-father-doctor directing and controlling the female-wife-mother-nurse in the interests of the child-patient. Subordination as a mode of domination in other words denoted a gender relationship. Midwives undoubtedly were easier to subordinate because they were women. Had they been men it seems more plausible that one of the other modes of domination would have resulted. Subordination thus reflects a patriarchal division of labour and relates closely to sexual and occupational divisions in the health workforce.

Yet the subordination of midwives cannot be viewed *just* as a process of male medical imperialism. As well as a gender transformation, a class transformation also took place. The rise to political and economic power by the medical profession was accompanied by the decline of other working class practitioners besides midwives, most particularly the so-called 'quacks' who were mainly men. Both class and gender are located within the social relations of production as relationships of domination and subordination.

A prime example of the interrelationship between class and gender is the strategy of creating lying-in hospitals. Working class females were used by middle class male-midwives to gain crucial knowledge in their overall struggle to control the occupation of midwifery. In fact, this control was more important than the 'knowledge' gained, as is attested to by strategies by which doctors in attendance at birth contrived to be 'fussily inactive' and to effect 'masterly inactivity' (ie doing nothing extremely well).

The question of the relative importance of class and gender I have argued varies with historical contingency. The subordination of midwifery to medicine analysed here has involved a complex interweaving of class and gender struggle without being ultimately reducible to either. As I have argued elsewhere, in collaboration with Johanna (Wyn) Willis, I am inclined to the view that in this instance gender struggle takes precedence. The gender aspect of this historical struggle is quite explicit; in the genderisation of medicine in 1862, the 'Sairey Gamp' ideology and the restrictive regulations of the 1915 Midwives Act. The process of medical subordination of midwifery may be seen as part of an historical 'struggle between male and female workers in which the better-organised male craft unions succeeded in overriding the interests of women workers' (Barrett, 1980: 165). Furthermore, the current sexual division of labour in health care was established *before* the advent of 'scientific knowledge'. This involved the alliance of male midwifery with surgery and the exclusion of women from formal medical and surgical training. The sexual division of labour thus provided the basis for the occupational division of labour.

6 The limitation of optometry

In this chapter the second principal mode of domination of health occupations by medicine, that of limitation will be analysed. Optometry is the occupation chosen to illustrate the operation of this mode. Limitation as a mode of domination of other health occupations by medicine has two principal characteristics. The first involves restriction of the occupational territory on which the occupation operates. This restriction may be to a specific part of the body (as is the case with dentistry) or to utilising a specific therapeutic technique (eg pharmacy). The second distinguishing feature of limitation is the relative independence of these occupations from medicine in the day-to-day administration of their activities. The independence is a relative one since medicine has usually retained an influence in the administration of these occupations through representation on registration boards. The limitation is spelt out in the registration Acts which specify exactly what constitutes the occupational territory of these occupations including techniques and diagnostic aids which may be used, while at the same time exempting medical practitioners from the provisions of the Acts. The Acts themselves have been the result of lengthy negotiations and struggles in which the lobbying of medicine has played a prominent part.

In the Australian health system those health occupations which exist in a relationship of limitation with medicine include dentistry, pharmacy, optometry, and more recently chiropractic and osteopathy. Other occupations such as physiotherapy are moving towards a relationship of limitation from one of subordination as they drop the referral requirement; that is they take patients for treatment without the necessity of referral by a medical practitioner.

From amongst these occupations optometry has been chosen in order to analyse the mode of limitation. The division of labour around the occupational territory of the eye is complex because several occupations overlap in their claims to occupational territory and thus compete for patients. The major struggle has been between optometry and ophthalmology, the result of which has been the limitation of optometry which is the focus of this chapter. It is the existence of ophthalmology as a specialised branch of medicine in the eye health service field which makes the analysis of optometry interesting. In order to understand the complex state of eye health services it is necessary to explain what health occupations are involved. These are as follows:

Ophthalmologists are medical practitioners who specialise in treatment of eye disease. Formerly called oculists they have specialist qualifications, either membership of the Royal Australian College of Ophthalmologists (henceforth RACO) or fellowship of the Royal Australian College of Surgeons in ophthalmology. A small proportion also do not belong to the colleges but are recognised by the Commonwealth Health Department for payment of specialist benefits as ophthalmologists. Being medical specialists, ophthalmologists obtain most of their patients through referral by general practitioners. Besides being specialists in medical and surgical treatment of eye disease and disorder, ophthalmologists also prescribe spectacles and other visual aids.

Optometrists basically solve vision problems that do not require surgery or chemotherapy. The exact definition of optometry has been a contentious issue and the statutory definition varies from state to state but basically the services provided by an optometrist

> are those of examination of the eyes and related structures to determine the presence of vision problems and other abnormalities; prescription and adaptation of lenses and other optical aids; the use of visual training aids to preserve or restore maximum visual efficiency and eye safety; and the supplying and services of prescribed optical aids. (Commonwealth Health Department, 1980: 208)

Formerly called opticians, optometrists are registered in all states of Australia although there is some variation between the various registration acts. Unlike ophthalmologists, optometrists do not have a direct channel of referral of patients to them. Optometrists are trained to detect and identify ocular pathology (eye manifestations of disease) but not to treat it. Referral of such cases to ophthalmologists for treatment is legally required. Optometrists are trained in a three to four year course in a tertiary institution.

Orthoptists are subordinated, working under medical supervision, usually that of ophthalmologists. They have no statutory registration but are registered with the Orthoptic Board, a subcommittee of the RACO. Ophthalmologists and orthoptists are represented on the board in the approximate ratio of two ophthalmologists for each orthoptist. Whereas opthalmologists and optometrists are overwhelmingly male, orthoptists are overwhelmingly female. The first orthoptists began in the United Kingdom after the First World War.

They were usually the daughters of ophthalmologists and assisted their fathers with training patients (especially children) in the correction of strabismus (squint) and in the measuring of visual fields. The first orthoptic clinic in Australia was begun in 1931 at the Alfred Hospital in Melbourne. Training was initially at the Eye and Ear Hospital but was transferred to three year tertiary level training in 1975. From being concerned primarily with visual field training, orthoptists have expanded their occupational territory to include other forms of investigation under medical supervision, particularly glaucoma. The crucial feature of the work of orthoptists is that they work only for ophthalmologists. It is a condition of their registration with the Orthoptists Board that they may not be employed by optometrists. It is a reflection of the extent of state patronised medical dominance that public funds are utilised to train an occupation, the employment and direction of which is the exclusive preserve of another occupational group.

Ophthalmic nurses are trained through post basic ophthalmic courses provided on an in-service basis by specialised eye hosptials for general registered nurses (Commonwealth Health Department, 1980: 189). In other words it is one of the specialised areas of nursing (such as midwifery, and intensive care) in which a general registered nurse can acquire training. Ophthalmic nurses assist generally in eye surgery and specialised care for patients with eye diseases and eye abnormalities. Being part of nursing, they are subordinated to medicine.

Optical dispensers interpret and dispense optical prescriptions and fit, repair and service optical appliances, principally spectacles. They may fill the prescriptions of either optometrists or ophthalmologists and may be employed by either although some run their own private optical dispensing businesses. Major optical dispensing firms such as Optical Prescriptions Spectacle Makers Ltd (OPSM), employ a significant proportion. They do not perform refractions nor 'offer opinions' on eye health, abnormalities or defects of sight (Commonwealth Health Department, 1980: 203). Training in most states is a two year course in a technical college and many are recruited from the ranks of optical mechanic tradesmen. There is no statutory registration and conditions under which optical dispensers practise vary considerably from state to state.

Optical mechanics are trade trained, serving apprenticeships of four to five years depending on the state. Their work involves 'surfacing, grinding, edging, calculating, making up and cutting out or fitting of prescription spectacles. In some instances it may also include the specialised activity of the manufacture of contact lenses' (Commonwealth Health Department, 1980: 206). Optical mechanics may be employed by either optometrists or optical dispensers. As indicated above many optical mechanics eventually progress to being optical dispensers by taking the relevant course. The process of the centralisation and concentration of capital has meant that many of them are employed in large scale organisations. The Australian Optometrical Association (AOA) estimated their numbers in 1974 to be about 900 (including apprentices) of which one firm, OPSM Ltd, employed more than 200 (Commonwealth Health Department, 1980: 207).

With so many occupations engaged in providing eye health services it is little wonder that the occupational territories overlap. Some of these are relatively minor. Optometrists for instance receive some training to enable them to do their own dispensing or 'jobbing' as it tends to be known. Yet most find it more convenient (and profitable) to send the work out to specialised optical dispensing firms. A few employ their own optical dispensers. Hence the phenomenon of pass-the-task or what Larkin (1981) calls 'sub-professional specialisation' has occurred within optometry as it has within ophthalmology where some tasks have been given over to othoptists. Ophthalmologists are not trained to dispense and so *must* send out their prescriptions to be made up by optical dispensers. This need has led to one of the important features of the eye care industry, the close relationship between opthalmology and one particular firm of optical dispensers, OPSM Ltd. The channelling of a large proportion of the prescriptions for spectacles from ophthalmologists to this one company has meant that it has come to dominate the lucrative optical dispensing market to an extent unparalleled in other countries.

Orthoptics is another task which comprises part of the occupational territory of both optometrists and orthoptists. However because orthoptists are subordinated to ophthalmologists most of the potential conflict between optometrists and orthoptists has been diverted to the major struggle of optometry with ophthalmology. The main area of dispute over occupational territory is the task of refraction or measuring the powers of vision which is hotly disputed despite the official limitation of optometry. Limitation this chapter will argue, is a mode of dominance involving compromise. Optometry has not been limited in a way which has fully satisfied medicine, but medical dominance has nonetheless been defended.

Eye health services involve four aspects: dispensing and sale of spectacles, diagnosis and measurement of refraction error, detection of eye disease, and treatment of these diseases by surgical or chemotherapeutic means. The first and last of these services are not disputed. The dispensing and sale of optical protheses is the acknowledged domain of the optometrist and the treatment of eye disease is the acknowledged domain of ophthalmology. This aspect of the division of labour in eye care services is a consequence of the limitation of optometry. In all registration acts of optometry, the treatment of eye disease by surgical or chemotherapeutic means is specifically excluded. The tasks which are contentious are the other services, eye examination for the presence of refractive errors and disease. Once the actual examination has been made it loses its contentiousness. If disease is detected the patient must be referred to an ophthalmologist for treatment. If no disease is detected however, the optometrist can proceed to test for refractive errors and prescribe and sell spectacles to the patient in order to correct these refractive errors. An ophthalmologist finding refractive errors writes a prescription for spectacles which the patient then takes away to be filled by an optical dispenser, often OPSM which may make rooms available for rent by opthalmologists so as to be able to offer dispensing facilities close by.

Hence the crux of the issue. Optometrists have been limited in the sense that they cannot treat the diseases of the eye they detect. Yet beyond that the issue becomes much more contentious. The major areas of disputation is the optometrist's competence to detect eye disease and the consequent danger or safety of patients attending optometrists for eye examinations. Optometrists' knowledge of ocular pathology and their consequent ability to adequately perform eye examinations is thus at the very centre of the issue to be discussed. The extent of the incidence of eye disease must be kept in perspective however. Epidemiological studies of the incidence of eye diseases in Australia have shown it to be only 1–2 per cent of the total population (Australian Bureau Statistics, 1975). In other words the overwhelming proportion of persons seeking eye care are likely to have healthy eyes and a visual problem which does not require medical attention.

The dispute is thus a relatively narrow one which has not much figured in public, despite persisting for more than 70 years. The account of the struggle to be presented here focuses mainly on the differences between the two occupations, but it is important to point out that a number of fairly basic similarities also exist. Optometry and ophthalmology share the same paradigm of 'scientific' medicine, they use the same instruments such as the ophthalmoscope (a device for examining the interior of the eye), the same terminology and prescribe the same sorts of spectacles. Some differences in technique exist but these do not appear to be major. Furthermore the struggle has not been between optometry and medicine as a whole, so much as with a specialised segment of medicine, ophthalmology.

The case of optometry is also somewhat different from the other limited health occuptions such as pharmacy and dentistry. The reasons for this are complex and historical and cannot be examined closely here but basically in neither the case of dentistry nor pharmacy has a medical specialty emerged which competes for the same occupational territory. In the case of dentistry, considerable autonomy was gained by dentists before medicine emerged in its present form. With pharmacy, the dispensing of drugs was a task delegated from the work of apothecaries when they were absorbed into medicine.

Outlined above then is the current division of labour in the eye care domain of health services. In order to understand the complex situation which exists today it is necessary to consider how it evolved into that situation. The process to be analysed then is a further instance of the reproduction of medical dominance. As with previous chapters I intend to analyse the evolution of the relationship between optometry and ophthalmology through a number of periods. The first two, the English antecedents and the Pioneer Era to 1911, provide the background for the major periods to be analysed concerning the emergence of optometry (1911-35) and its professionalisation and legitimation (1935-73). The process to be analysed is the emergence of optometry as a distinct occuption, its shedding of a trade background and adoption of a strategy of professionalisation in its attempt to gain autonomy, a secure niche in the health division of labour, and collective upward social mobility for its members. Again the focus is primarily upon Victoria although at times it has been necessary to discuss events occurring in other states.

The debate has been a highly technical one and no attempt is made to judge the technical issues involved. Rather the emphasis is upon differences between therapists of various sorts and the occupational associations set up to represent them. A further difficulty experienced has been the bitterness associated with the struggle, not only between medicine and optometry but also within optometry itself. My interest in these conflicts is not at the level of the personalities involved but at the more structural level, and in particular to the extent that they represented different processes in the reproduction of medical dominance on one hand and different strategies for the professionalisation of optometry on the other.

English antecedents

Opinion differs as to who first invented spectacles. Roger Bacon, the English philosopher-scientist and monk of the thirteenth century is usually credited with the discovery, although the Chinese contribution is not altogether clear and may have preceded Bacon (Gasson: 1980). What is known is that the use of spectacles dates from about the fourteenth century. The invention of printing in the fifteenth century appears to have given a further impetus to spectacle making which began along trade lines. The extent of literacy however was relatively small and spectacles were expensive to produce so their use was confined to the affluent.

In 1629 King Charles I granted the charter to the Worshipful Company of Spectacle Makers which gave them power to regulate the trade (Champness, 1952: 4). For about 200 years after that the guild was active in exercising their powers, policing inferior work and regulating the occupation. Optical and mathematical instrument makers also sold spectacles, the latter belonging to the Watchmakers Company. In 1756 the title 'optician' appears for the first time in the company's records. By the end of the eighteenth century it appears the 'optician' had emerged from the spectacle—making trade. By the end of the nineteenth century opticiantry had become divided into opthalmic opticians who tested sight and prescribed spectacles; and dispensing opticians who filled those prescriptions. This division continues to the present day in the United Kingdom and provided the basis for the differentiation between optometrists and optical dispensers in Australia. At the end of the nineteenth century 'sight-testing opticans' in the United Kingdom were of three main types. A minority were medically and surgically qualified, the majority were trained by apprenticeship and the third group were totally untrained (Fielding and Portwood, 1980: 36).

In discussing the antecedents of eye care services prior to the development of Australian society it is important to relate the development in the use of spectacles to the political economy of the time. Prior to the industrial revolution the use of spectacles was limited to those who were literate and wealthy. The mass of the rural based non-literate agricultural population had little use for or indeed means of acquiring spectacles. The transition from feudalism to capitalism dramatically changed the importance of vision care in the health services of the society. On one hand industrial methods became available for the production of lenses and frames which greatly reduced their individual production costs. On the other hand, early industrial capitalism in its 'laissez-faire' stage made almost impossible demands upon a mass scale on people's capacity for close vision work. What had been adequate for agriculturally based feudal society in terms of visual ability was no longer so in a factory based capitalist system with poor lighting, for the required indoor labour, long hours of close precision work and later extensive reading.

A high level of visual ability on a mass scale was thus important. Without it the expansion of industrial production would have been limited by the natural visual ability of the majority of individuals. The development of visual aids and their refinements was thus important to the development of capitalism and could be said to be one of the benefits flowing from it, though working conditions of early captialism took an enormous toll of eye as well as general health. The foundations were laid for improvements in visual ability associated with leisure activities such as driving, movies and television in the twentieth century. Another factor which spurred the development of spectacles was increasing longevity. With a larger proportion of the population reaching 65 years of age, when almost 100 per cent require spectacles for presbyopia (old age long sightedness) the demand for spectacles was much greater and spurred the development of innovations such as bifocals.

The development of *ophthalmology* as a medical specialty is associated with the evolution of medicine in general, a topic which is examined in an earlier chapter. Ophthalmic surgery, the crux of ophthalmology, began during the eighteen century but according to the major figure in ophthalmology in the twentieth century, Sir Stewart Duke-Elder (1957), was considered an unimportant and unrewarding side issue for general surgeons. In 1805 Moorfields Hospital was established in London for treating diseases of the eye, the first such special hospital in the world.

The major boost however came in the mid-nineteenth century at the time of major new discoveries that revolutionised medical science and led to the emergence of the germ theory of disease and the paradigm of scientific medicine. The invention of the ophthalmoscope by Helmholtz in 1850 in particular, allowed the examination of the interior of the eye and provided the technological foundation for the establishment of ophthalmology as a specialised part of medicine. Whereas clinical ophthalmology had been chiefly surgical, the ophthalmoscope 'expanded the subject of disease of the eye beyond the confines of surgery by confronting the ophthalmologist with the field of fundal pathology and its intimate relation to general medicine' (Rosen, 1944: 24).

Medical specialties can be classified into four types; some deal with specific age groups (paediatrics, gerontology), some with certain technical procedures (radiologist), some dealing with certain organs and organ systems (orthopaedists, ear, nose and throat, etc). Ophthalmology although having its origins in the utilisation of a specific procedure—ophthalmoscopy (use of the ophthalmoscope)—quickly became one of the fourth type, dealing with a certain organ, the eye. In terms of the complementary processes of segmentation and accretion by which specialties appear, outlined previously, the case of ophthalmology Rosen (1944: 4) argues, is a clear instance of accretion and segmentation operating sequentially. Accretion occurred with the splitting away of ocular surgery from general surgery drawing in those interested from the fields of pathology and general medicine. Segmentation has subsequently occurred with the splitting away of ophthalmology from ENT (ear, nose and throat) to form a separate specialty. While technological advances such as the invention of the ophthalmoscope were important, most historical accounts tend to reify that technology. As an earlier chapter argued, it is necessary to examine the social context in which those technological advances occurred and the social relations which made their utilisation possible. The emergence of a new medical specialty was the result not only of the production of the new technology itself. As was argued in an earlier chapter drawing on the work of Peterson (1978), the early development of specialisms can be seen more as a form of medical entrepreneurship than the result of technological innovation or the desire for research. Specialising resulted in benefits not so much in economic terms directly but in terms of connections and visibility.

In order for that technology to appear and exercise influence Rosen argues, two other factors must be present. The first of these is the rise and propagation of the concept of *feasibility*, that it is feasible for the back of the eye to be seen. Thus a 'sense of problem' which derived from the new paradigm of scientific medicine, was of crucial importance. The 'sense of problem' is also important for the second factor as well; the recognition of the importance of that discovery and the transmission and diffusion of that information to other medical groups by writing and teaching.

Rosen and Peterson both argue that ophthalmology was one of the first of the specialties to emerge and its arrival was viewed with hostility and suspicion by the mass of the profession who often saw it as a form of commercialism. The improved knowledge and specialised techniques, and their use by doctors furthermore does not necessarily constitute a specialty, Rosen (1944: 36) argues. 'A number of men operating within a limited field of practice do not constitute a specialty which can only be said to exist when there are bonds between practitioners, bonds which take shape within an association based upon like interests and common problems.' On this criterion, ophthalmology can be said to have existed as a medical specialty in the United Kingdom since 1880, the date of the formation of the Ophthalmological Society of the United Kingdom (Duke-Elder, 1957: 27).

That ophthalmologists were treating eye disease by the last decades of the nineteenth century there is no doubt. When they began testing vision and prescribing glasses is less certain. It has been claimed in the United States for instance that refractions were conducted by ophthalmologists from the start (American Medical Association, 1961: 495) but there is little evidence to support this contention. In Duke-Elder's (1957) account of the history of ophthalmology for instance it is significant that no mention is made of refraction as part of the work of ophthalmologists. It seems more likely that ophthalmology's interest in refraction is of more recent origin and that some of the advances in the techniques of vision testing and the techniques associated with it, would have been made by opticians.

Thus far I have analysed the origins and early development of optometry and ophthalmology up until about the beginning of the twentieth century. This has been necessary as background in order to understand the early development of the two occupations in the Australian, particularly Victorian, context which is the subject of the next section.

The pioneer era

The first reference to an oculist in Victoria is in 1855 when one Samuel Jacob practised in Elizabeth Street, Melbourne (Melbourne Commercial Directory 1855). The 'father of ophthalmology in Australasia' (Williams, 1947: 9), JT Rudall arrived in Melbourne in 1858, bringing an ophthalmoscope with him. Williams credits Rudall along with Gray and Bowen as having established ophthalmology in Australia. In 1863 Andrew Gray founded a charitable infirmary for the treatment of diseases of the eyes and ears of the poor, located in Albert Street, Melbourne. It was the first specialist hosptial to be established in Australia and it is Melbourne's third oldest hospital (Gardner, 1968). In 1870 this institution became amalgamated with another specialised eye benevolent institution 'The Ophthalmic and Orthopedic Institution', which had been established by T Aubrey Bowen in 1869. In 1873, it was renamed the 'Victorian Eye and Ear Hospital' wit!. Bowen and Gray as honorary surgeons.

During the latter decades of the nineteenth century there was a small but active number of oculists practising but the specialty of ophthalmology only gradually became established. As the Melbourne hospitals developed they appointed specialists to their staff and oculists were often the first to be appointed, as Bowen was to the Children's Hospital in 1873. It was a further eighteen years before another specialist of any other type was appointed (Lowe, 1980).

Dissemination and diffusion of new technical information was also brought about by Australians travelling to the United Kingdom for specialised study in eye diseases, usually at Moorfields Hospital in London and then disseminating this information to their local colleagues on their return. Edward Gault for instance, qualified in medicine at Melbourne University in 1890, travelled to London to study at Moorfields Hospital in 1892 and returned to practise in Melbourne about 1895, becoming the honorary surgeon to the eye department at the Alfred Hospital after a short stint in general practice (Lowe, 1980). Moorfields remained the mecca for aspiring Australian ophthalmologists at least until specialised training became available in the 1930s in Australia. In this way the developments in ophthalmology made by the major European figures such as Donders and Van Graefe were disseminated locally.

Yet as Rosen as indicated, a number of men operating within a limited field of practice does not constitute a specialty and ophthalmology may be said to have emerged only with the development of bonds between the practitioners in the formation of the Ophthalmological Society in 1899. The Ophthalmological Society was based on its United Kingdom counterpart which had been formed in 1880. Three of the founders of the Ophthalmological Society of Melbourne were members of the British Ophthalmological Society, having joined during visits to London. The five Melbourne surgeons who attended the inaugural meeting were all recognised as specialists in disease not only of the eye but also the ear and throat.

Meetings were held for seven years until 1906 when the society disintegrated through lack of interest. It was not until after the present period (1912) that a society was reformed, this time not as a separate specialist society but as the Eye, Ear and Throat Section of the British Medical Association (Lowe, 1980). In 1938 this became the Ophthalmological Society of Australia (with other state BMA sections). In 1969 the Australian College of Ophthalmologists was formed and in 1977 the 'Royal' prefix was added to become to RACO. To say that ophthalmology had fully emerged during this period then is premature. While there were surgeons with special interests which included the eye as well as the ear and throat, the segmentation and accretion process necessary to the formation of a medical specialty had only partially occurred. The other point to be made is that the interest in ophthalmology was wholly directed at eye disease. At the various medical congresses which were held from 1887, papers on eye subjects were quite common (sixteen at the Congress of 1899) though very few of these dealt with the issue of sight testing (Williams, 1947).

Whereas quite good records exist of early oculists this is not the case with opticians. Histories are written mainly about the middle and upper classes and the working class, from whence opticians originated, have received little historical treatment. The 1855 *Melbourne Commercial Directory* mentions one optician—W Abrahams. The Sands and Kenny *Melbourne Directory* of 1857 lists three opticians practising in and around Melbourne. Anyone could call themselves an optician and their practice consisted mainly of importing and selling ready made-up spectacles. Hence the practice of 'choosing' a pair of spectacles, ie by trial and error until a suitable pair were found. Travelling hawkers and peddlars usually supplied the visual needs of the rural population, taking a box of ready made-up glasses on their travels to sell with their other wares.

In this era there appears to have been little competition between oculists and optometrists, and as far as can be ascertained fairly harmonious relationships seem to have existed between the two occupations. Like ophthalmology, optometry had not fully developed its own occupational identity. The division which developed in the

United Kingdom between ophthalmic opticians (sight testers) and dispensing opticians (optical dispensers) was not yet developed in Australia and it was common for optical supply companies to offer the sight testing part of the transaction 'free', charging only for the sale of spectacles. Indeed the first training in optometry in New South Wales appears to have been carried out by optical supply companies who sold 'trial cases'; offering a two week rudimentary course in optics to train the buyer to use the case.

In general though entry into optometry was by one of two means. Younger entrants usually did an apprenticeship with an established practitioner, while 'mature age' entrants did a tutorship course. One such tutorial system was that offered privately in Melbourne by Mr Henri Van Heems from about 1900. The course consisted of twelve lessons and cost five guineas (Aitken, pers. comm.). In 1904 a Sydney optometrist, H Sanderson stimulated the first attempt at an occupational association for optometrists. The Australasian Optical Association was a national association including New Zealand optometrists and by 1906 had 53 members. The attempt proved too ambitious for the times however, given transport and other difficulties. Separate state associations were formed instead. Charles Wright (1980a: 145), the AOA historian, suggests that the reason for its formation was the growing tension between optometry and ophthalmology.

It was formed because the ophthalmologists had started blackballing optometrists in a joint association which then existed. Ophthalmologists had no difficulty relating to optometrists as unorganised individuals but about that time optometrists were beginning to work towards legislative recognition as an independent primary profession.

During the pioneer era then both ophthalmology and optometry had their Australian beginnings though neither had a distinct occupational identity by the end of the period under consideration. Of the two, ophthalmology was better developed, though its attention was concentrated more upon diseases of the eye than upon refraction. Ophthalmology also tended to be associated with ear and throat disease as well. Optometrists for their part were largely untrained and most of their work consisted of the sale of ready made-up spectacles, often in conjunction with other occupations such as jeweller, pharmacist or hawker.

Having examined the background to the professionalisation of optometry and its struggle with ophthalmology, the first of the major periods to be analysed concerns the emergence of optometry in the period 1911–1935. The second concerns its professionalisation and legitimation in the period 1936–1973.

The emergence of optometry 1911–1935

In 1911 the Victorian Optical Association (VOA) was established, an occupational association which set optometry firmly on the professionalisation road. The VOA set about achieving 'closure' of optometry through the dual strategy of education and legislation. In conjunction with this it set about 'putting its house in order' by seeking to emulate the model of professionalisation provided by dentistry. The position of dentistry within the health division of labour, as one of what might be called 'acceptable limitation' (ie largely accepted by medicine), was much envied by optometry and its leaders on a number of important junctures had the dentistry model of professionalisation firmly in mind. That optometry has not achieved 'acceptable limitation' even today is the process to be analysed. The professionalisation of optometry was not fully achieved by 1935, that date is chosen as the date optometrists achieved statutory registration and hence regulation in Victoria.

The VOA began with six members. As few practising optometrists of the time had any formal education in optometry (apart from a few graduates of English optometrical training courses), the criteria of qualifying for membership had to be established. The VOA operated its own 'grandfather clause' to achieve this, setting eligibility as having practised as a refractionist for two years if a principal (ie in charge or sole practice), or three years if an assistant. Travelling or itinerant vendors of spectacles (defined as having no fixed place of business) were specifically excluded. Hence from the start optometrists set about pursuing a strategy of closure by excluding those considered undesirable and unbecoming of its aspirant professional image. At the same time, efforts were made to secure recruitment from across different classes with the low educational entrance required (Merit Certificate taken after eight years of schooling), night and correspondence courses.

The primary initial thrust of the VOA however was in the field of education. In 1912 a course of study was introduced (based on the model of the British Optical Association) leading towards a Fellowship of the VOA (FVOA). This became the professional qualification until 1943. From the start there was some difficulty in arranging lectures in specific subjects through tertiary institutions. The Pharmacy College was tried, Melbourne University approached, unsuccessfully due to the recommendation of the medical faculty (Minutes, 4, 1926: 430); until arrangements were made with the Melbourne Technical College from 1930 (Gray, 1940: 291–292).

The second prong of the professionalisation strategy related to regulating the conditions of practise for optometrists and promoting the emergence of optometry with a distinct occupational identity.

Important in this strategy for all occupational groups has been the publication of a journal to provide information to members. Journals act as a basis for unifying the occupation as well as disseminating and transmitting specialised knowledge. Until 1911 the journals that existed reflected the nature of optometry at the time, catering to the chemist-optician and jeweller-optician. The *Australian Manufacturing Jewellers, Watchmakers and Opticians Gazette* (henceforth AMJWOG) for instance, had a regular 'optical notes' column and was the official organ of the VOA until 1918. In 1911 the first specialised optometrical journal was published, eventually to become the *Commonwealth Optometrist* on the formation of the Australian Optometrical Association in 1918. At the same meeting, a resolution was passed, asking states which supported a supplement in *trade* journals to 'discontinue the practice' (Kett, 1953: 15). By cutting loose from its trade origins optometry began actively to pursue a strategy of professionalisation.

The nature and organisation of optometrical work did not change it is important to note, but the occupational ideology certainly did. The ideology of professionalism began to be espoused as optometry sought to abandon its trade connotations. Such an ideology was imitative of dentistry and ultimately medicine itself. Victorian optometrists had to be reminded of this in 1923 when a jewellery trade paper offered VOA members cash prizes for articles on optometry. An editorial in the *Commonwealth Optometrist* (Oct., 1923: 162) argued '... we feel sure that Victorian optometrical essayists will need no invitation to support their own *professional* paper in preference to that of the Jewellery *Trade*' (emphasis added).

In fact what was beginning to emerge at this time was a division within optometry which has remained important up until the present day. The work of the optometrist consisted of two parts: testing vision and selling spectacles. The first part falls easily within the range of conventional health services, the second does not, but falls more within the commercial sphere. A tension arose within optometry as to which part of the optometrist's service was the most important. Those who argued the vision testing part stressed the professional model of development, while those stressing the selling aspect advocated a commercial model. Hence a division emerged which has been important to the development of optometry along professional versus commercial lines.

The issue which most clearly reflects this tension is that of advertising. The 'professionals' aspiring to the occupational model provided by medicine and dentistry favoured the limitation of advertising. The 'commercials' by contrast regarded advertising as a normal and legitimate business activity. Particular concern was expressed however at what was considered unethical advertising. The fourth AOA conference in 1921 discussed this practice by 'uncontrollable practitioners' concluding 'this festering sore was appreciated as a great hindrance to professional optometry' (Kett, 1953: 18). It was seen as a hindrance because advertising (on trams, billboards etc) promoted a model of optometrists as primarily sellers of spectacles with the sight testing of minor importance.

The professionals on the other hand stressed the skill necessary to test sight as the crucial aspect of a professional optometrist's practice. Some commercial optometrists offered the sight testing part 'free' in order to attract customers, an anathema to the professionals who strongly opposed the practice. The first conference of the AOA in 1918, passed a resolution urging optometrists to discontinue the practice (AMJWOG, Dec., 1919: 44). In 1924 the VOA asked its members to give a written undertaking not to indulge in the practice and many did. In 1925 the rules of the VOA were changed to prohibit *advertising* that sight testing was free. A vote taken amongst members however, showed how widespread was the practice with almost half the members, revealing they made no charge (Commonwealth Optometrist, July 1925: 124).

In pursuit of the professionalisation strategy, a code of ethics was adopted by the AOA conference in 1921 and spelt out the duties of optometrists to the rest of the profession and to the public (Kett, 1953). Several practices of a more commercial nature which had been the subject of criticism were forbidden in the code of ethics. These included exaggerating the patient's visual defect so that a sale of spectacles could be made and promising results to be attained by use of spectacles. It also spelt out conditions under which referral to an oculist should be made (any sign of eye disease). It enjoined optometrists not to criticise the medical profession or their prescriptions when dispensing but to endeavour to work in harmony. Finally, in the commercial sphere it oppposed house-to-house canvassing for patients, publication of fees and prices, and free sight testing. On advertising, a compromise appears to have been reached, it suggested that: 'all printed and displayed advertising of whatever form should be dignified and educational, expressed in good English and free from all extravagance and exaggeration' (A Code of Ethics for the Optometrical Profession in Australia, 1921).

Some of these ethical injunctions were obviously aimed at placating medical opposition to optometry in the hope of gaining status and legitimacy. The effect it should be noted was 'voluntary' limitation, the optometrists themselves played an active role in limiting their own occupational territory. Such a point is important since it shows that medical dominance operates in part at least through the voluntary actions of other occupational groups within the health division of labour. The effort of optometry in other words was directed more towards gaining legitimacy than achieving complete autonomy.

Through the period under consideration then, the VOA gradually tightened control over its members. Membership could be revoked for 'unethical conduct' in 1924, the grandfather clause for membership abandoned and passing an examination made the means of entry, prohibition on advertising discounts was made in 1933. All these actions outlined above constituted strategies in the professionalisation of optometry. All were attempts to regulate the practice of optometrists, to encourage and cajole the diverse individuals who called themselves opticians to conform to standards of practice which would lead to upward social mobility for optometrists.

Another important aspect of the professionalisation strategy was the promotion of a distinct occupational identity. The establishment of a specialised journal of optometry was one part of this. Another was the resolution of the VOA in 1919 to adopt the term optometrist rather than optician (Commonwealth Optometrist, 1.3.1919: 2). This is important for two reasons. Firstly it marked a move away from the British model of development which had been important unt' 'hat date. British opticianry as already indicated, had two parts: ophthalmic opticians and dispensing opticians. Wishing to establish a separate identity from the optical dispensers, the VOA chose an American word 'optometrist' which had come into use during the late nineteenth century and had been adopted by the American Optical Association in 1903. Secondly it reflected a strong claim to the occupational territory of vision testing. The instrument used for determining eye defects at that time was called an optometer and the science of using that instrument optometry. Hence adopting the designation optometrist both provided differentiation from the optical dispenser and strengthened the claim to the occupational territory of sight testing.

Yet all the internal regulation which optometry attempted was only partially effective while there was no control over who could designate themselves an optometrist. While this situation persisted anyone could do so and the reputation of the emerging profession it was claimed suffered from the activities of these 'quacks'. The need for regulation through statutory registration was recognised from the outset by the VOA and constituted its main activity from 1911 until 1935 when legislation finally was realised.

Certainly from the optometrists point of view regulation was sorely needed. What brought optometry into disrepute more than anything else was the commercial practice of using travellers or canvassers to generate business. Without statutory registration, the VOA was powerless to stop the frequently unscrupulous canvassers who travelled house-to-house either selling ready-made spectacles or securing appointments for an optometrist to call in order to conduct a vision test. This problem was particularly acute in the rural areas and working class areas of Melbourne. In one of the many deputations to see the Chief Secretary to lobby for legislation the problem of the rural areas was discussed. The president of the VOA, Mr Cumberland produced advertisements such as 'Baker, Pastry Cook and Optician', and 'Plumber, Gasfitter; sight testing a specialty' (CSO, 22/H8618, 30.8.1922). Another case cited involved a hawker selling women's clothing: 'He said he always took a case of spectacles with him on his travels and sold quite a lot. These were the cheapest spectacles at 18/– a dozen yet he admitted selling three pairs to a family and receiving six guineas.' (CSO, 19/E5677, 8.6.1921).

Reports of court cases in October 1912 demonstrate the seedier, commercial side of optometry of the day. In one of these for example the optician sued unsuccessfully for the cost of glasses provided. The defendant, a Richmond woman, explained,

> a hawker had called and asked if she suffered from headaches. She told him she did and plaintiff [the optometrist] came later and tested her eyes. He brought the glasses and got her to sign a paper without telling her how much they would cost. She signed and he then said 'The glasses will cost £2–10s'. Witness said she could not afford it and he told her she would have to pay because she had signed the paper. She did not wear the glasses and gave them to her sister-in-law to return. (AMJWOG, Oct., 1912: 34).

The woman also revealed in evidence that her husband earned only 30 shillings a week so the cost of the spectacles was one and a half times their weekly income. The case was dismissed. The extent of the use of canvassers is indicated by the fact that some optometrists actually advertised that they did not employ them and did sight testing at their rooms only.

Attempts by optometrists to secure registration legislation however had the effect of spurring ophthalmology into a more oppositional position and 1911 also marks the beginning of serious conflict between the two occupations in Victoria. The ninth congress of the Australian Medical Association in Sydney in 1911 was notable for the emergence of the Section of Ophthalmology under the presidency of the Melbourne oculist, James Barrett. The congress passed a special resolution; that in the public interest no legislation should be introduced which suggested that optometrists be legally authorised to test vision (Williams, 1947: 25). The congress did support subordination however, suggesting that opticians should be properly trained as spectacle makers so they could adequately fill the prescriptions of oculists and be subordinated to them as pharmacists were. '... the relationship of the optician and the oculist should be that of a pharmaceutical chemist to the physician.' (Optical News, 1911: 1)

The basis of ophthalmology's opposition to optometry at that time was the denial of optometrists competence to sight test adequately and hence a rejection of optometry's claim to sight testing as its occupational territory. That ophthalmologists treated eye disease and optometrists dispensed spectacles there was no dispute. The area between those two activities however was the contentious one.

In the ophthalmologist's justification of their claim that optometrists were not competent to adequately test sight, the elements of the ideology of professionalism were made quite explicit. Firstly ophthalmologists argued that only those who had medical training were competent to test sight since refraction was a medical procedure. The eye was not a separate optical instrument it was argued, 'but a living and inseparable part of the human body, sharing its diseases and consequently defects of vision are so frequently connected with conditions of local and general disease that their meaning and nature can only be properly ascertained by persons who have received a medical and surgical training' (VPD, 198, 22.10.1935: 3721).

Their claim that refraction was a medical procedure was strengthened by the argument that the use of drugs was necessary in order to adequately test vision. Medical orthodoxy of the time required the use of a drug called atropine which was put in the eyes to paralyse the ability of the eye to accommodate during testing. Optometrists could not legally prescribe and use drugs hence oculists argued it was impossible for them to adequately sight test and the optometrists' 'eye testing must be of a very crude character' (VPP, 2, 1914: 276). Because optometrists did not have the expert knowledge to test sight adequately oculists argued, they should not be registered as such. 'The sphere of treatment even by glasses was essentially that of the medical man and was outside their competence.' (AMJ, 23.8.1913: 1183)

The ophthalmologists strategy then was to claim a medical model for refractive errors, and by fusing eye disease treatment and measurement of refractive errors justify the exclusion of optometrists. On this basis the ophthalmologists justified their claim to the occupational territory of sight testing. A report of the Medical Advisory Board to the Minister of Public Instruction in 1914 argued: 'Eye testing they [the Advisory Board] consider is the work of the oculist and the oculist alone.' (VPP, 2, 1914: 276) Thirdly oculists opposed the more commercial aspects of optometry.

> It was now generally known by the public that headaches were often caused by errors of refraction and might be relieved by the wearing of spectacles. Opticians everyday advertised this fact and invited sufferers to go to their parlours for relief. Once seated in the optician's chair they never failed to buy a pair of spectacles and if the first did not relieve they purchased a second or a third ... (VPP, 2, 1914: 1181–1183)

Underlying this opposition was a quite clear economic fear of competition. 'The Bill really proposed to create a close corporation of
opticians who might keep to themselves a very lucrative trade under
the specious plea that it was a highly skilled profession.' (VPP, 2,
1914: 1183)

Finally there were class elements which underlay the opposition to
optometrists. Emphasis was made wherever possible of the optical
trade as against the medical *profession*. For instance in a deputation
to the Chief Secretary, a leading oculist Dr E L Gault claimed, 'So far
as the optician is concerned as a guild of skilled trained workmen they
have our great respect but when they aspire to the rank of professional
medical men we must tell them they can only qualify by the same
course as we have done' (CSO, 19/A 7889). In order to be adequately
trained to dispense the prescriptions of oculists, 'a boy entering the
trade should have some general education' (Kenny, 1920: 260), and
should be trained not in the university where more prestigious occupations are trained, but in a technical college. For all these reasons it was
claimed optometrists should not be registered as sight testers.

Optometrists responded with counter-arguments on each of the
arguments raised. Their main arguments was to separate treatment of
eye disease from sight testing. They agreed with the necessity of
medical training to diagnose and treat eye disease but not to test sight
since sight testing was not a medical procedure, arguing '. . . measuring the powers of vision is no more an essential part of medicine than
the making of a boot for a misformed foot' (Cumberland, CSO,
19/E5677, 8.6.1921). Similarly, optometrists claimed the use of
optical instruments was not the preserve of one occupational group
(Bell, CSO, 19/E4677, 8.6.1921).

While optometrists accepted that the treatment of eye disease was
the occupational territory of the ophthalmologists, they did lay claim
to being able to detect eye disease and refer patients on to ophthalmologists. Hence the ophthalmologists' claim that they did not have
medical training, optometrists argued, did not prevent them being
able to adequately test sight. In order to be able to detect disease
however they needed training in ocular pathology and this need
became probably the major source of contention in later years.

To the claim that the use of drugs was necessary to adequately test
vision, optometrists argued that the use of atropine was unnecessary
in order to competently test the powers of vision. Their 'limitation' to
the non-use of drugs in other words was not seen as a problem, since
they claimed their use unnecessary. To support their contention they
were able to cite several leading American oculists. History furthermore has revealed their correctness and the ideological nature of the
doctors claims. Atropine is rarely used to assist refraction nowadays
and is certainly no longer part of medical orthodoxy. The use of
atropine therefore provided a strategy for differentiating the sight

testing performed by oculists from that performed by optometrists. Since only oculists could legally use atropine, and its use was claimed by them to be essential, then by implication only oculists could adequately test the powers of vision. Oculists claim to the occupational territory of sight testing would be strengthened as a result. On the claims of commercialism the optometrists argued it was a type of 'Catch-22' situation. The reason why registration was desired was precisely so that the more blatant commercialism of some optometrists could be controlled. It was the lack of registration which permitted such advertising to occur. Optometrists also denied that spectacles were prescribed unnecessarily or that mercenary motives were uppermost.

In all, optometrists denied the oculists claim to sight testing as their occupational territory, citing historical precedent of the oculists becoming concerned with sight testing and spectacle prescription as a comparatively recent concern. The claims and counter-claims which emerged during this period have provided the basis for the conflict which has continued up until the present day.

Gaining statutory recognition and registration was a principal aim of the VOA from the outset in 1911. By early 1913, the VOA had prepared a draft bill 'for the Registration of Sight-Testing Opticians' and met with the Acting Premier, Mr Murray, in June to press for its introduction into Parliament (AMJWOG, Aug., 1913: 24–28).

As we have seen the Opthalmological Society reformed itself in 1912 and became the Eye, Ear and Throat Section of the BMA early in 1913 (Lowe, 1980: 264). A special meeting of this body was called in mid-June to discuss the proposed bill. Strong opposition was expressed to the proposal to register opticians as sight testers. The meeting was 'in hearty accord with any and every attempt to expand the education and training of spectacle makers and opticians but we cannot approve of state legal recognition of sight testing by spectacle maters since this is most certainly a part of the practise of medicine' (Minutes, Eye, Ear and Throat Section, BMA (Vict)).

A controversy ensued involving deputations to senior politicians, correspondence in the newspapers, and pamphlets to members of parliament. A meeting of the oculists on 25 November was urged by the secretary 'to do some active work among the members of parliament in order that the bill might be effectively stopped' (Minutes, Eye, Ear and Throat Section . . . , Nov., 1913). The bill came before Parliament in November under the title 'Opticians Act' with the support of the Acting Premier (VPD, 20.11.1913: 2625). It reached a second reading before the government, defeated on another issue, went out of office and the bill lapsed. The minutes of the Eye and Ear Section of their March, 1914 meeting leaves little doubt of the reasons for the optometrists lack of success:

... the temporary defeat of the Bill was largely due to the uniting efforts of the Hon. Secretary Mr Leonard Mitchell seconded by the willing help of each and all of the members. *If the ophthalmic surgeons of Australia could stick together as the Melbourne ones had done he had no doubt as to the fate of any similar bill.* (Emphasis added, Minutes, Eye, Ear and Throat Section ..., Jan., 1914)

However 1913 marked only the beginning of a 22-year struggle by the optometrists to gain registration and regulation of their occupation. Throughout this time they were opposed by the ophthalmologists who continued in their attempt to subordinate as much as possible or at the very least deny it legitimacy in the sight testing area. Limitation *per se* seemed to have been largely taken for granted. There was no suggestion at any time that optometrists should begin treating eye disease or that they should cease practise altogether. Rather the struggle was over the *extent* of limitation to be imposed on optometry in exchange for legitimation by the BMA and the state.

Deputations from both sides met with government representatives on numerous occasions between 1913 and 1924 but a similar impasse resulted. The government changed in 1924 and Sir Stanly Argyle, a medically trained parliamentarian who has figured in previous chapters became Chief Secretary and attempted to arrange a compromise. It is obvious from the record of the deputations that the oculists were by this time becoming somewhat isolated within the larger BMA, as there appeared to be considerable support from within the BMA as a whole for a bill to register opticians (CSO, 24/M5974, 19.5.1924). Oculists constituted only one segment of medicine and while most doctors probably felt some obligation towards colleague solidarity, the struggle with optometrists tended to be seen (and still is) as a fairly narrow sectional struggle which did not greatly affect the rest of medicine. Apathy from the bulk of the profession has long been one of the thorns in the side of ophthalmology.

In the mid-1920s a new argument in favour of registration was introduced. This had been achieved in Tasmania in 1913, Queensland in 1917 and South Australia in 1920. The effect of these acts on Victoria it was claimed would be that all the 'quacks' who could not get registration in those states would travel to Victoria to continue their practices (CSO, 24/M5974, 19.5.1924). Legislation in New South Wales in 1930 added further weight to this argument. Yet legislation could still not be agreed upon. Argyle was keen to see a bill passed but was unwilling to do so without the agreement of his medical colleagues. He argued,

... the eyesight of the community is a most important thing. Many businesses and trades cannot be carried on by people with impaired eyesight. It is most essential that the eyesight of certain employees in the railways department, of pilots and of other men who have to navigate ships should be all right. We should prevent ill informed persons, with nothing but their impudence to recommend them practising on people and endangering their eyesight. (VPD, 170, 19.11.1925: 2266–2267)

Throughout the period from 1913 to 1934 then the opposition of the ophthalmologists to registration of optometrists as sight testers would appear to be the major reason why legislation was not forthcoming. Indeed the ophthalmologist were given an assurance in 1920 that the government would not take any action unless the opticians could come to an agreement with practicing ophthalmologists (MJA, 18.9.1920: 261). The dominance of medicine's expertise within the health division of labour was sustained and its opposition prevented the legitimation of optometry.

Yet a contradictory aspect of ophthalmology's argument became increasingly apparent. Having failed to subordinate optometry, it attempted to limit its occupational territory severely. While recognising that opticians would not abandon sight testing, ophthalmologists argued that *no one* should be registered specifically to test sight. Market forces then would ensure the bulk of the work going to ophthalmologists. 'The public will soon recognise the higher class of work (performed by ophthalmologists) and an increased demand will call for an increased supply of highly skilled ophthalmologists.' (MJA, 18.9.1920: 261) Hence ophthalmology would come to dominate the sight-testing market. However lack of registration also had the effect of permitting 'open slather' in sight testing so that anyone could perform it.

Relations between optometry and ophthalmology developed at levels other than the legislative one in the period 1913–1934, and were predominantly characterised by a hardening of attitude on the part of ophthalmology. The area of contention which emerged in this era and which has continued until the present day, concerned testing the eyesight of children. The ophthalmologists sought to preserve this area for themselves, arguing at various stages that sight testing of children by optometrists should be banned in any legislation to be passed. State patronage for medicine ensured that sight defects detected by school medical officers would be sent to oculists though an early government report found in 1914 that although Melbourne was well served by oculists, only three of the large country towns had an oculist available for refractive work. Hence ophthalmology's attempt to secure this area of work was limited by the lack of oculists available to do the considerable amount of work involved (VPD, 2, 1914). The AOA conference of 1925 expressed strong opposition to this discrimination against optometrists (Kett, 1953: 19).

On the ophthalmological side an important event in 1932 was the formation of Optical Prescriptions Spectacle Makers Ltd (OPSM). One of the difficulties that ophthalmologist faced in the struggle over the occupational territory of sight testing was their reliance on opticians to actually dispense the spectacles from the prescriptions written by ophthalmologists. Before the separation in optometry occurred between those who just dispensed (in English terms dispensing opticians) and those who also tested sight (ophthalmic opticians), ophthalmologists had little choice but to send their prescriptions to optometrists. Many ophthalmologists believed in addition, that optometrists were charging excessively for prescription-only services, thus discouraging patients from consulting ophthalmologists. In the earlier part of this era as we have seen, while subordination of optometrists was still sought it was suggested to ophthalmologists they patronise optometrists (with their prescriptions) who would agree not to do sight testing. John Nathan, a Collins Street optometrist whose father Bert Nathan was a major figure in the development of optometry (the chairman of the first registration board), recalls that his father was approached by several ophthalmologists in the early 1930s offering to send him all their prescription work (ie an assured supply of business) if he would give up sight testing. Bert Nathan declined the offer but it was taken up by another.

In 1932 OPSM was formed in Sydney specifically to fill the prescriptions of ophthalmologists and *not* those of optometrists. The extent of ophthalmological involvement in the establishment of OPSM has been the subject of allegations and speculation but little is known and considerable secrecy surrounds the firm. A recent article of investigative journalism by Sydney optometrist/journalist Ralph Lewis (1978), examines the development of OPSM in detail. The secrecy was necessary Lewis argues, because the founder Gordon Champion (himself an optician), held several agencies for the supply of optical goods to wholesalers, who then supplied them to optometrists. Had his involvement become known the optometrists' power of boycott of his products would have ruined his business. The source of the original operating capital for the company is not known according to Lewis, though there is evidence that a leading Sydney ophthalmologist, Dr Darcy Williams was involved and that its formation was a specific strategy in the struggle with optometry (AMA Gazette, Oct., 1982: 35). OPSM set up near the practices of ophthalmologists (originally in Macquarie Street) and its convenience and lower prices attracted considerable business whether prescriptions were directed by ophthalmologists or not.

OPSM quite soon began to affect optometrists who responded in two ways. Firstly they attempted to find who was behind OPSM and Lewis reports stories of Gordon Champion being followed around the city. Secondly they threatened to close their accounts with wholesalers who supplied OPSM. Both of these were unsuccessful and OPSM has gone from strength to strength to become one of Australia's largest companies today. The establishment of OPSM was important in strengthening the position of ophthalmology because it enabled the 'colonisation' of two new areas of business. Whereas ophthalmologists had been concentrated in the 'specialist' areas of big cities (Macquarie Street, Collins Street), they were able to expand into suburban areas as the company provided dispensing facilities wherever ophthalamologists chose to practise. They also provided assistance, such as advice to young ophthalmologists setting up in business.

The other areas of colonisation was in the 'intermediate' level of eye care services, traditionally the major source of the optometrists work. Ophthalmologists private consultation fee in 1930 was two guineas (about $50 by modern standards) (Lewis, 1978). As such their services were restricted to the affluent. 'Intermediate clinics' were set up in Melbourne and Sydney to provide a lower cost service. In Melbourne the clinic was known as the 'Medical Eye Service of Victoria'. OPSM held the dispensing contract (ie supplied the spectacles prescribed) and the service was staffed by younger and semi-retired ophthalmologists. General practitioners were encouraged to refer their poor patients there for vision testing. Both clinics became popular and a considerable source of business and income was denied to optometrists. OPSM has made generous contributions to ophthalmological causes and has also been important in referring patients to ophthalmologists. The relationship between OPSM and ophthalmology has been a highly successful one and reduced the work of optometrists considerably, especially in New South Wales.

The effect of OPSM in Victoria did not take long to be felt by both the commercial and professional segments of optometry, each of which by 1934 had its own organisation. The Master Opticians Society (MOA) represented the commercial segment and consisted mainly of employers of optometrists, that is principals in the larger more commercially oriented optometrical firms which had by this time emerged. The professional strand was represented by the VOA. The MOA responded to the establishment of OPSM in Victoria with emergency meetings to discuss the 'threat' of 'uncompetitive cut prices offered to the public by the medically supported cut price house' (AMJWOG, Aug., 1935: 29). The threat to the livelihoods of both 'commercial' and 'professional' optometrists acted as a powerful force for unity and papered over the tension between the two segments which otherwise divided them. The need for legislation was seen as urgent. Without registration the ability of optometrists to compete adequately with organisations like OPSM was severely reduced. The MOA had previously been hesitant about the idea of registration as they feared it would increase the cost of employing optometrists to work in their business.

The optical supply houses (the wholesalers) were also threatened by ophthalmology's expansion and joined forces with the optometrists in an attempt to secure legislation. As the *Gazette* commented, 1935 was probably the first occasion that the full optometric and optical resources of the state had been brought to bear on a single objective (AMJWOG, Sept., 1935: 29). A legislative committee was formed with representatives from the VOA, MOA and the wholesalers and a 'fighting fund' begun to finance the activities of the committee. This was raised by a tax on optometrists' monthly accounts with wholesalers and the wholesalers themselves contributed a proportion of their turnover. A lobbyist was hired, Mr W Gray who had been involved in optometrists' campaign against OPSM in New South Wales and South Australia. Gray organised another conference with the oculists but agreement still could not be reached (Gray, 1940: 292). Then an intensive campaign of lobbying politicians began which included the discreet passing of contributions from the fighting fund to the coffers of the government party (Nathan, 1980: 164). Support for the bill was secured amongst all parties and the bill was introduced into Parliament in October, 1935. The BMA circularised members arguing against the bill and the medical lobby in Parliament introduced two 'hostile' amendments to the bill in an attempt to change it. One proposed equal numbers of optometrists and medical practitioners on the Optometrical Registration Board and the other proposed that optometrists should not be allowed to treat anyone under the age of eighteen. After further intensive lobbying both these amendments were defeated (VPD, 198, 22.10.1935: 3734).

The important amendment which was made however, was one which allowed advertising by optometrists. Despite their unity in opposing ophthalmology, the commerical and professional tension reemerged over the issue of advertising. The professionals, pursuing the model of professionalisation provided by both medicine and dentistry, wanted a ban on advertising. The commercials however, in particular the large Melbourne firm of Coles and Garrard supported the retention of the right to advertise as a basic business right and crucial to competing with firms such as OPSM. With the support of some members of parliament in particular the Labor leader of the Opposition, Mr J Cain, the clause which had originally allowed the board full control over advertising was amended. To the 'professional' faction it was quite clearly the price of achieving legislation.

... unfortunately after the second reading of the act we were faced with an alternative of accepting the present clause or loosing the support of the [word missing in transcript] a party which at that juncture meant no act. After very serious consideration the committee decided that the act could always be reopened at a later date and it would be better to accept the condition that loose [sic] the bill. (B Nathan files)

The influence of the commerical faction can be seen further by the fact that the two government appointees to the registration board were, for a considerable period, representatives from the large commercial firms, especially Coles and Garrard. The clause permitting advertising remained a source of contention until the 1970s. An enigmatic editorial in the *Journal of Optometry* (20.12.1935: 590) argued in reference to the clause that 'optometry has been shot at by arrows feathered from its own wings'.

The bill was passed early in December 1935 and passed into law, ending more than two decades of struggle by optometry. The bill had been passed against the wishes of the ophthalmologists within the BMA and nominally at least the BMA as a whole. Many medical practitioners it appears accepted the inevitability of eventual registration for optometrists. The dominant position of medicine was hardly threatened by the bill either. The act did not forbid sight testing by unqualified practitioners but did statutorily restrict the term optician. Optometry was 'limited' in its statutory definition to using methods for measuring the powers of vision other than those which involved the use of drugs. It was also 'limited' to sight testing and spectacle provision and not the treatment of eye disease. Of the seven members of the board, two were to be medical practitioners nominated by the BMA. The other five were to be opticians, two nominated by the government and three by the opticians themselves. Hence optometry was also 'limited' by having medical representation on its registration board. Medical practitioners were exempted from all provisions of the act of course. The grandfather clause (section 8) was set at five years; that is a person had to have been practising optometry for not less than five years prior to the act to qualify for registration. Persons who had practised optometry for between three and five years were eligible for registration subject to passing an examination. In the first register published in 1937, 168 of the 286 optometrists registered (59 per cent) qualified under this clause (VGG, 22, 27.1.1937).

One other clause was particularly important to the professionalisation of optometry. It gave the board autonomy to police the act and the conduct of optometry by allowing deregistration under certain conditions including 'infamous conduct in any professional aspect'. As we have seen previously, the attainment of this clause by medicine was important in the production of medical dominance. Because the term 'infamous conduct' was undefined, it gave the board consider-

able power to ensure that individuals follow the policies by the professional association. Thus by the end of the period under consideration
statutory registration had been achieved by the optometrists, even in
the face of opposition from ophthalmologists, though at the price of
limitation. Victoria was one of the last states to do so in fact. The
effect of registration was to set optometry firmly on the professionalisation path although it did little to diminish the opposition of ophthalmology; opposition that manifested itself in many ways during the
next period.

Professionalisation and legitimation 1936–1973

In this period I propose to trace the further development of optometry
following registration and the continuing dispute with ophthalmology. Registration meant 'closure' of the occupation. It limited the
use of the occupational title 'optometrist' and 'optician' to those
registered under the act. Once that was achieved then the other major
thrust of the professionalisation strategy could be implemented; that
of setting up an appropriate course of study to ensure higher
standards of practice through minimum competency for all optometrists. In other words once control over the occupation itself was
achieved then similar control could be pursued over who became an
optometrist. The educational reform of optometry was crucial its professionalisation and also the main means of political advancement vis-
a-vis ophthalmology.

Under the act the Optometrical Registration Board (ORB) was
empowered to institute a training course for future optometrists. Its
attempts to do this in consultation with Melbourne University raised
again the long standing controversy over the teaching of ocular
pathology to optometrical students which had begun as early as 1921.
In order to strengthen their claim that sight testing and eye disease
treatment could be separated, the optometrists argued they could
detect the presence of eye disease (not diagnose or treat) and refer
patients to ophthalmologists for treatment. In order to detect ocular
pathology however they needed training in the subject, training which
could only feasibly be provided by ophthalmologists. Not surprisingly
ophthalmology has been reluctant to teach ocular pathology to
optometrists and thus undermine its own claim to the occupational
territory. In 1921, the Eye, Ear and Throat Section of the BMA has
refused a request from the VOA for lectures on eye disease resolving
that 'it considers that a knowledge of diseases of the eye is not
necessary to the training of an optician' (Minutes, Eye, Ear and
Throat Section ..., April, 1921).

The ORB met with the (Melbourne) University Extension Board
and a four year course of study was drawn up involving basic science

subjects in early years and specific optometrical ones in later years. The proposed curriculum was considered by a joint committee of the Faculties of Medicine and Science who reported back in March 1937. Their report was critical of that part of the curriculum dealing with pathological conditions on the eye claiming it would give optometrists a smattering of medicine. It suggested a two year course of instruction with only elementary instruction in the anatomy and physiology of the eye, claiming that training in general pathology and medicine had nothing to do with optometry (Medicine Faculty Minutes, 5, 1938: 459–460). In an endeavour to get the training programme underway approaches were made to the Melbourne Technical College but this was strongly opposed from within the VOA as likely to lead to a lower status profession and one unlikely to be able to compete socially and politically with university trained doctors and dentists. Plans were drawn up for the creation of an Australian College of Optometry (ACO) to train optometrical students, modelled along the lines of the Dental College. Further negotiations with the university led to an arrangement whereby optometrical students could take their first two years of their training in the university doing basic science subjects and then the latter two years in the college, training in specialised optometrical subjects.

The college opened in 1940 with a total of eighteen students, thirteen of whom were inherited from the old VOA course, and Judge Stretton as its first president. The college trained and examined students for the Licentiate in Optometric Science (LOSC) which became the registrable qualification. One of the issues which concerned the council early was what entrance requirements to expect of students. Medicine and dentistry had 'matriculation' (the right to enter university) as their entry standard but there was concern amongst some optometrists about the difficulty in attracting students if the entry standard was set that high (Gray, 1940: 292).

The driving force behind the creation of the college and first chairman of the council which administered it was Ernest Jabara. He had previously argued strongly against training at the Melbourne Technical School, claiming that it was a submatriculation institution more suited to the training of tradesmen. Professionals he argued, were trained in universities and thus 'matriculation' had to be the entrance standard. Jabara stressed dentistry as the occupational model which optometry should follow. In an influential paper, reprinted in the *Australasian Journal of Optometry* (1941b), he argued that the different experiences of two other health occupations had clear lessons for optometry. Massage, which had achieved registration in 1923 had been subordinated to medicine. Dentistry on the other hand was a much more suitable model ('a shining example') of occupational development.

Jabara was later the figure around whom a major split occurred in the ACO in 1942. While personality clashes and the commercial/ professional tension played an important role, there were also ideological differences involved. One of these was a difference in what constituted the science of optometry. Jabara, American influenced, stressed optometry as an applied *biological* science while the more traditional English view tended to see optometry as a more *physical* and mathematical science and one which had developed through the discipline of physics (Jabara, 1941a: 435–453). The controversy was important to the development of optometry as it set the direction of development for the next twenty years or so. It was largely between what might be called 'visionaries' and the 'pragmatists'. The 'visionaries' subsequently withdrew from all participation in the college but it is noteworthy that most of their ideas were subsequently realised at a later date. While Jabara undoubtedly pushed his colleagues too far too fast along the professionalisation road, the framework was laid for subsequent realisation of his aims, at a later time considered more appropriate. One example of this was that the original consitution of the college specifically allowed for affiliation with the university even though this did not occur until twenty years later (Gray, 1940: 294).

The first (five) students began training in 1941 at the university in basic science subjects including physiology. From the outset the difficulty was in receiving adequate clinical instruction in physiology, especially of the eye. Because of the lack of clinical material, a meeting of the board with university representatives in November 1942 resolved to ask the Ophthalmological Society (OS) to provide an ophthalmologist to lecture and demonstrate to optometrical students at the Eye and Ear Hospital in the means of internally examining the eye to detect disease known as ophthalmoscopy (B Nathan Files). Two years of correspondence and meetings ensued without the OS agreeing to cooperate and the issue became deadlocked.

As 1943 progressed the matter began to come to a head. The Act had empowered the ORB to draw up an optometrical curriculum and the refusal by ophthalmology to assist in providing tuition in a part of the curriculum could be seen as obstructing the will of Parliament. The Chief Secretary entered into the dispute and attempted to coerce the opthalmologists into providing instruction. Their response was to threaten to withdraw their services from the Eye and Ear Hospital, a course of action unheard of in the 1940s. By this time however, notice of the disunity within optometry had come to the Chief Secretary's attention and that coupled with the strike threat led him to back down (B Nathan Files; also Williams, 1954: 32–33). Soon after the responsibility for the administration of the Act was passed from the Chief Secretary's office to the Hospitals and Charities Commission.

The attitude of the OS hardened after this and a third condition for their cooperation was communicated to the ORB in November. They resolved 'that the Ophthalmological Society considers orthoptics is a method of treatment and therefore the society is insistent that the act be amended to forbid its practise as a necessary condition to its cooperation in the instruction of optometrical students in ophthalmoscopy' (Correspondence, B Nathan Files, 1944). The occupation of orthoptics was emerging under medical control and ophthalmology laid claim to this occupational territory as their own. The claim was rejected by the ORB who claimed orthoptics was accepted as part of the occupational territory of optometry in English speaking countries (B Nathan Files, 1945).

The struggle ended in a stalemate. In the meantime however, the ACO had found a way around the ban during 1943. It had advertised for an ophthalmologist to teach optometrical students and had succeeded in attracting Collins Street ophthalmologist, Dr R L Naylor, to provide instruction in ocular pathology from 1944. Naylor, who is reported to have been unpopular with his ophthalmological colleagues before accepting the appointment was not prepared to accede to pressure from the OS for no ophthalmologist to accept the post, nor to relinquish it. While he could provide lectures however, access to clinical material was still denied optometrical students. This state of affairs has continued to the present day with optometrical students still receiving no clinical instruction at the Eye and Ear Hospital and this lack of clinical training remains something of a deficiency in the training of optometrists.

The struggle however demonstrates the strength of feeling in this particular demarcation dispute. Ophthalmology was able to use its considerable political power to defeat attempts to coerce it, even though it could be seen to be obstructing the will of the people expressed in optometric legislation. The opposition to teaching optometrical students has been formalised into a ban as one of the rules of RACO and continues to the present. Even if individual ophthalmologists were favourably disposed towards teaching or addressing optometrists the strict enforcement of this rule and denial of permission operates as a powerful sanction.

Two other aspects of optometry's professionalisation deserve mention here since they both are concerned with the attempt to legitimate optometry in the wider sphere. The first of these is the official recognition of optometry at the main annual Australian scientific congress in 1939. AOA delegates successfully argued for the inclusion of the 'subject of optometry' in the physics section of the Australian and New Zealand Association for the Advancement of Science (ANZAAS) conference in Canberra (Wright, 1980: 4). Recognition secured considerable scientific legitimacy for optometry which could be translated into political advantage.

The second aspect was the voluntary enlistment of optometrists in ophthalmic units in the Australian Armed Forces during the Second World War. The debate over relative rank for optometrists and ophthalmologists is an interesting microcosm of the long struggle between the two professions. With medical domination of the army medical corps the inclusion of optometrists was not a rapid event. Indeed it took two years of negotiations before an officer status was secured for optometrists and in May 1942 the first optometrists were commissioned with the rank of lieutenant (Kett, 1953: 30). Optometry was recognised as an essential public health service and its members exempt from war service except as volunteers. Optometrists were also appointed to wartime bodies set up by the Commonwealth. Such acts helped to secure the politico-legal legitimation of optometry. Ophthalmologists, to the disappointment of many, received the rank of major (two above that of optometrists) (Williams, 1953: 23). Actually one very beneficial consequence resulted from the wartime experience, that optometrists and ophthalmologists worked together for the first time and many developed a better appreciation of the work of the other.

The major feature of this period besides educational advancement however was optometry's incorporation into the National Health Service, again against the wishes of ophthalmology. As we have seen in previous chapters, from the beginning of the twentieth century, the state began to take a greater role in the provision of health services for its citizens. Whereas under 'laissez-faire' capitalism the distrbution of health resources had been left to market forces, with the development of capitalism the state began to intervene in the market place in an attempt to ensure a more equitable distribution of health resources. The possibility of a national health scheme spurred the reactivation of the AOA in 1937 and a special committee was appointed to deal with the issue of national health (Kett, 1953: 30). The issue was temporarily shelved by the government during the Second World War but a special meeting of the AOA in Melbourne in 1942 met to discuss the National Health Scheme. The thinking of the government at that time was towards a full-time salaried service and the AOA prepared a scheme for optometry to fit into this. Later when government thinking veered towards a part-time service, a second scheme for the inclusion of optometry was prepared. Both schemes retained the right of private practice for individual optometrists. The story of the attempts to introduce a national health scheme has been told elsewhere (Hunter, 1969) but neither scheme was ever introduced.

In 1948 the Optometrical Services Committee was formed by the AOA to negotiate the inclusion of optometry into any national health scheme. The Health Minister of the time, Sir Earl Page (a medical practitioner himself) proposed that a Commonwealth benefit should be paid for eye examinations but only when that examination was carried out by an ophthalmologist. A government subsidy would have made ophthalmologists considerably cheaper than optometrists and seriously affected optometrists share of the eye examinations performed. The optometrists directed their lobbying at the Prime Minister, RG Menzies. Menzies overruled Page and prohibited the payment of a Commonwealth benefit for a medical examination at which glasses were prescribed. This became the notorious section 4.4 of the National Health Act of 1952. Rather than include optometry in the National Health Scheme, a course of action the government was not prepared to take, ophthalmology was excluded from a subsidy on the task which was disputed. Hence in theory neither optometry nor ophthalmology would have a competitive advantage. The decision was a setback for ophthalmologists as they became the only medical specialty for whom a basic part of their work did not attract a health insurance benefit.

In practice however, a way to circumvent the intention of this section fo the Act was soon discovered. Through their influence in the private health insurance funds, an 'ancillary' benefit was made available to the patients of ophthalmologists which compensated for the lack of a government benefit. Other means to circumvent the spirit of the Act were also developed but the effect was to give the ophthalmologists a substantial advantage. At least 75 per cent of the fee paid to an ophthalmologist could be recovered by various means. This fact, coupled with the close relationship with the dispensing firm OPSM, meant that ophthalmology increased its share of the primary eye care market from about 10 per cent in 1952 to about 30–35 per cent by 1972 (Wright, 1979: 204). In that time also the number of practising ophthalmologists quadrupled. The AOA complained bitterly about what they saw as an anomalous situation of discrimination but achieved nothing until 1972 when a federal Labor government, under EG Whitlam, came to power. Part of Labor's election platform was a promise to introduce a universal health scheme and it immediately established a number of review and investigatory commissions. A further period of intense submission writing and lobbying resulted, the optometrists side being conducted principally by the AOA Executive Director, Dr Damien Smith. The importance of the negotiations was not lost on Dr Smith and the AOA Executive. Failure to gain inclusion in what became called Medibank would have been the death of optometry as a clinical profession (pers. comm. Dr Damien Smith). Through 1973 and 1974 the meetings and lobbying continued with ophthalmologists again arguing for the subordination of optometry, suggesting that the general practitioner should act as the 'portal of entry' for optometrical services as he or she did for other medical services. The general practitioner should decide whether to refer patients on to optometrists for a refraction to be done. To cut a long story short, the government announced in May 1974 that optometrists were to be included in the proposed universal health care scheme (Medibank) as primary contact practitioners, an event which occurred in 1975. The optometrical negotiators shrewdly held out a carrot to the government of a 'participating agreement' on fees. Optometrists offered to guarantee that they would not charge more than the fee scheduled by the government for services provided. The advantage to the government was in terms of a precedent which it hoped (to no avail) other medical groups, in particular medicine, would follow. Such an agreement would constitute a means of containing cost increases. The price of some government regulation was greater legitimacy in all respects and there is no evidence optometry has since regretted the arrangement.

1973 was also an important year in Victorian optometry as it marked the full admission of the Department of Optometry into the University of Melbourne within the Faculty of Science. In 1958 the first full-time lecturer, Mr Barry Cole, was appointed to the college. In 1961 an agreement was reached with the university for the college to become part of the newly created Faculty of Applied Science. The optometrical training course now became the Bachelors Degree in Applied Science. In 1968 optometry was transferred to the Faculty of Science and the qualification became a Bachelors Degree in Science (Optometry). Finally, the University Department of Optometry was established in 1973 (Wright, 1979: 112).

In universities which have medical schools, the medical faculties are invariably powerful and active in university politics. Given this fact it may seem unusual that optometry could again entry and remain in a university setting. This it was able to do even in the face of recommendations that it be moved. The Martin Report on the Future of Tertiary Education in Australia in 1964 for instance recommended that the training received in optometry should be decanted off to a college of advanced education. Several reasons would seem to explain this, notably considerable support from powerful university figures, an active policy of research, but most importantly there appeared to be little evidence of medical faculty opposition to the incorporation of optometry into the university. The segmentation of medicine is thus important in explaining the professional advancement of optometry in the period under consideration. Apart from ophthalmologists who were in direct economic competition with optometrists, the rest of the medical profession, especially those in the academic institution felt little threat from optometry.

While the main focus of this analysis ceases in 1973, in the period since 1973 one or two issues are important as they mark the culmination of a long process. The first of these is the continuing tension between the 'commercial' and 'professional' sections of optometry.

The professionals have gradually gained control over advertising since registration. In 1946 changes to the regulations banned a number of what were considered objectionable commercial practices including door-to-door canvassing, paying commissions to agents for introducing patients, and misleading advertising (VGG, 3.7.1946: 2). Finally in 1975 'window displays' of spectacle frames in the window of optometrists' offices were more controlled when it became a condition of membership not to do so. However the move was a contentious one. A poll amongst members of the AOA in Victoria revealed almost a third of optometrists were opposed to such a change. As a result it was decided not to incorporate the ban into the regulations of the board, altering only the code of ethics.

The second event of importance to the evolution of optometry was a move against the 'limitation' which had been imposed upon it. With growing legitimacy, the profession obviously felt confident to do so. A more militant leadership also seems to have been a factor. In 1975 the act was amended to remove the two medical practitioners from the registration board. The board then became comprised entirely of optometrists. The other initiative was against the limitation on optometry in the use of the certain sorts of drugs. Optometry in the original 1935 act had been defined as measurement of vision without drugs. During the 1960s however there was a gradual move toward overcoming this limitation, particularly in New South Wales. In Victoria a de facto situation has arisen which allows optometrists to utilise certain drugs for specific purposes, especially dilating the pupil. Optometrists have permission to use some restricted drugs under the Pharmaceutical Act and while they cannot legally use these to refract they can be used to dilate.

The explanation given thus far in the chapter tends to relate mainly to 'official' relations between optometry and ophthalmology, that is at the level of their professional associations. Relations at the individual level may be quite different. In the academic sphere in particular where there is no competition between the two professions there is considerable cooperation and quite friendly relationships. In the Low Vision Clinic at the Royal Victorian Institute for the Blind, for instance, academics from both occupations cooperate and share clinical facilities. Joint research projects have been carried out and the senior academic ophthalmologist, Professor Gerard Crock, has supervised the post-graduate research of some optometrical students.

In the private practice sphere there are some friendly relationships between optometrists and ophthalmologists, especially in a concentrated area such as Collins Street, where there is a high density of optometrists and ophthalmologists. Many optometrists develop referral relationships with special ophthalmologists for those patients where eye disease is detected. However the economic competition for patients between the two professions acts as a barrier to their effective cooperation.

Another recent move in the direction of better relations between optometry and ophthalmology has been a change in the policy of OPSM. From about 1973, OPSM began to move away from such a close affiliation with ophthalmology. Optometrists were employed by the company, the ban on filling the prescriptions of optometrists was lifted and the 'setting up in practice' service extended to optometrists. This is not to imply any particular altruism on the part of OPSM. The decision would appear to have been influenced by the prospect of optometry gaining entry into Medibank and hence receiving a greater share of the market, as well as legal advice as to the possible consequences of the Trade Practices Act. The decision to employ optometrists would appear to be based on a desire to exploit the lucrative contact lenses area. This new development became largely the occupational territory of optometry because of the need for training in optics and the importance of the fitting of the lenses; neither of which ophthalmology undertakes.

At the official level however the dispute continues and looks likely to continue to do so in the foreseeable future. The RACO for instance, recently employed a former New South Wales Premier, Sir Eric Willis, to give the organisation more political clout. There have also been several instances of leading optometrical academics having offers of research paper presentation or even attendance at ophthalmological conferences refused (pers. comm., Dr Barry Collin).

The process of limitation

In the development of optometry two models of occupational organisation were available to follow: one along professional lines and the other along commercial business lines. The differences between the two should not be over-emphasised however. Both are private enterprise entrepreneurial activities conducted in the market place. The difference is principally the ideology of professionalism which claims a different rationale for the same commercial activity. Both the commercial and professional models developed alongside each other with considerable tension manifesting itself at various times, especially over the issue of advertising.

Indeed the tensions have been such that had it not been for medical opposition to both factions acting to unify optometry, it would probably have split into two separate occupations at some stages of its development (notably in 1935 and 1974–1975). An important factor in the professionalisation of optometry then has paradoxically been medical opposition itself. Attempting to overcome this opposition has been an important stimulus to professionalisation. Major benefits have accrued from professional organisation however, in legitimacy, status, and ultimately economic terms. But while medicine was unable to prevent the legitimation of optometry, it was able to 'limit' its occupational territory and thus leave professional dominance largely unchallenged, at least until the 1970s. Paradoxically had medicine, in particular ophthalmology pursued a different strategy towards optometry the subordination of optometry would have been likely. Had ophthalmology not claimed sight testing as its occupational territory then as state intervention in the health system increased, optometry would quite likely have been put 'on referral', as the National Health System developed. Attendance at an optometrist in other words would most likely have been made conditional upon referral from a medical practitioner. This would have placed optometry in a structural position similar to physiotherapy, or indeed orthoptics. By pursuing sight testing as its occupational territory, ophthalmology bought into a struggle in which it did not lose, but did not really win either, and limitation was the result.

'Limitation' is thus basically a mode of domination involving compromise. As such it is a form of restricted recognition. Ophthalmologists it appears would have preferred the subordination of optometry or at least its exclusion from the occupational territory of sight testing. It was unsuccessful however, partially it appears because support from medicine as a whole to press for subordination or exclusion was not forthcoming. Yet medical dominance in the division of labour has secured considerable political advantages for ophthalmology in its relation with the state. The School Medical Service and the Repatriation Department both utilise the services only of ophthalmologists, much to the chagrin of optometry.

Optometry pursued the professionalisation model provided by dentistry and medicine in its development. However in one crucial respect it differs markedly from that model in the existence of the right to advertise commercially. What the eye care field of health reveals in a fairly naked form is the capitalist organisation of medicine. In no other area of health care is consumer choice such an important aspect. Lenses correct vision defects but the choice of a spectacle frame involves a fashion element. The cosmetic effect of spectacles has long been recognised and links health care with fashion probably more than in any other area of health service provision. Spectacle frames can be purchased for about $25–$30, yet patients pay up to $150 for a spectacle frame (pers. comm. Mr Daryl Guest, AOA). The difference between the basic cost and the actual cost is called the 'fashion component' and is huge.

This difference has implications for the mode of domination experienced by optometry, since a part of its occupational territory is clearly non-medical although mixed with 'medical' procedures. Medicine's interest has been in limiting those medical aspects as much as possible and this aim of controlling only an aspect of optometrists' practices helps explain why limitation rather than some other mode is experienced by optometry.

A further feature of the limitation of optometry suggested by the analysis is its inherent instability. The struggle, particularly since 1935 has mainly been optometry pushing, with considerable success, against the limitations imposed upon it. The instability of limitation I would argue in this case results from the overlapping occupational territories of the two occupations concerned. There is a parallel body of practice within medicine, in contrast to other 'limited' occupations such as dentistry where there is not, and where limitation is more stable as a result.

The analysis here however should not be taken to mean that medical dominance is particularly threatened by the legitimation of optometry. As Larkin (1981) argues in his analysis of the same struggle in the United Kingdom, the legitimation of optometry alters the terms rather than the substance of the medical dominance. Despite state recognition of optometry the process of limiting occupational autonomy within health care to doctors (what I have called the production and reproduction of medical dominance) has continued. What the empirical example of ophthalmologists and optometrists reveals indeed is the dynamic rather than static form which the production and reproduction of medical dominance takes.

7   The exclusion of chiropractic

The third mode of domination of other health occupations by medicine is exclusion. As a feature of the reproduction of medical dominance some occupations within the broader health division of labour have been excluded from official recognition within the health system, have no registration and no state supported education or subsidised treatment through insurance rebates. These occupations collectively have come to be known under the umbrella term of 'alternative' health care. This label is a consequence of their exclusion which is part chosen and part imposed. They exist outside the conventional medical division of labour, forming instead a part of the much broader health division of labour. These occupations include osteopathy, chiropractic, naturopathy and acupuncture.

Historically these 'alternative' modes of health care have had varied careers. Homeopathy for instance, as was analysed in a previous chapter, has largely withered away. Some occupations now within the conventional medical framework, such as physiotherapy, began as 'alternative' modes but have been incorporated. Amongst all of them however chiropractice has stood out as the most persistent and successful, and has flourished despite its exclusion. This chapter analyses chiropractic and its relationship with medicine, both at the level of their knowledges about healing and of their practitioners. First the emergence of chiropractic as a distinct health occupation in the United States is analysed prior to practitioners of chiropractic arriving in Australia. Then its development and professionalisation in Australia, especially Victoria, is considered with particular emphasis on its attempts to secure legitimation and a secure position in the health division of labour. All this occurred in the face of considerable medical opposition to its very existence.

The process of legitimation is thus a central concern; legitimation of both a body of knowledge and an occupation based upon that knowledge. The conflict with medicine in this process is usefully viewed as a power struggle, one aimed at securing an occupational territory upon which to practise.

The process is analysed through until 1978, when chiropractors achieved substantial legitimation through a registration bill passed in that year in the state of Victoria. This makes the end of the official exclusion of chiropractic and a change in its structural position within the health division of labour to one more closely approximating limitation. Chiropractic has historically been excluded therefore and on that basis has been chosen for the analysis here.

The relationship between medicine and chiropractic has been a particularly stormy one. Scotton (1974: 23) for instance likens it to 'a holy war between the forces of good and evil'. It is still evolving furthermore with continuing hostility between the parties involved. As with the instances already examined, the conflict here is founded on disputed occupational territories. In the case of chiropractors the claimed occupational territory is more a technique than a part of the body. The focus is upon the spine, yet it is the technique of manipulation, or 'adjustment' in chiropractic terminology that is the basis of its claim to a position within the division of labour—that is, spinal manipulative therapy (hereafter SMT), the manual mobilisation of the joints of the vertebral column.

Now manipulation itself is by no means exclusive to chiropractic; indeed that has been a major obstacle to its legitimation. As we will see, manipulation has been an important therapeutic technique for centuries, having originated with bonesetters. Chiropractic (along with osteopathy) is the only occupation to focus and utilise it *exclusively* for healing purposes. Manipulation is used by both medicine and physiotherapy—the major opponents of chiropractic—hence the competition for occupational territory.

Manipulation in medical therapy occupies a paradoxical position. On one hand there is a small proportion of doctors who practise manipulation and advocate its wider utilisation. This group has usually been the most active against chiropractors. Yet despite its determined advocacy by supporters such as Cyriax (1973), manipulation is not widely utilised by medicine or physiotherapy and much of the medical profession remains skeptical of it. Even within medicine it retains the status of unorthodoxy which it has had since the days of bonesetters. Amongst physiotherapists also, training in spinal manipulation dates back only to about 1963, and while there are now manipulative therapy groups active in Victoria, it tends to have a specialised status. Most adherents, the Federal Committee of Inquiry into Chiropractic, Osteopathy, Homeopathy and Naturopathy (hereafter the Webb Report, 1977) found were in private practice and the ethic of referral from medical practitioners was often only a token gesture. Its use in physiotheraphy is more limited than in chiropractic; it tends to be palliative rather than curative in focusing on local relief rather than cure. It is bounded furthermore by a greater number of contra-indications (reasons why it shouldn't be used) than chiropractic.

How then is chiropractic different? As such it seems in terms of the theory on which it is based as in terms of the actual technique itself. The different terminology it appears has been specifically developed to reflect the difference in the knowledge upon which medicine and chiropractic are based. Initially this was to provide a defence for chiropractors against the charge that they were practising medicine. Medicine and chiropractic are thus different theories of knowledge about the origins of ill health and appropriate therapy. This is reflected in a number of ways. Both medicine and chiropractic use X-rays as a major diagnostic aid but in examining the X-rays a chiropractor may see subluxations whereas an orthopaedic surgeon does not. The extent to which these two theories of health knowledge are commensurable then is an open question. Medicine, as part of its political campaign against chiropractic, has tended to stress the incommensurability of chiropractic theory with 'scientific medicine', claiming that 'If the chiropractic concept is accepted then it must be assumed that the whole basis of scientific medicine as built up over the past two centuries by a vast amount of research and clinical investigation is fallacious' (AMA Report on Chiropractic, 1966).

The perceived incommensurability of chiropractic with medicine, it will be argued, has been the major factor which has dictated the use of exclusion as the mode of domination experienced by chiropractic. In its evolution, chiropractic ran into medical dominance of the health division of labour. Chiropractic began prior to the achievement of this medical dominance but was well established by the time it began to emerge seriously as a competitor in the period of expansion of medical dominance. This dominance furthermore was translated into medical sovereignty. The medical profession achieved state patronage, a form of delegated authority to control the health system. This as we have seen in a previous chapter was the result partially of class forces (backgrounds of doctors, etc) and partially the compatibility between the ideology of medicine and dominant class interests. This latter compatibility was associated with the corporatist mode of medical production as an earlier chapter indicated. It was also strengthened considerably by the ideology of professionalism—in this case that only doctors were competent to judge health matters since only they had the necessary expertise. Chiropractic however has continued to be characterised largely by the individualist mode of medical production. It tends to be labour rather than capital intensive, is diffuse, non-hospital based and stresses clinical experience. Such an approach to healing is a result of exclusion.

These factors are important in outlining exclusion as a mode of domination. As chapter two argued, medicine coopted the legitimacy of science and scientific legitimacy became fused with politico-legal legitimacy. Occupations which did not have scientific legitimacy could be excluded and described as a 'cult'. For this reason as this chapter will argue there was no question of statutory recognition of chiropractic (unproven as it was) and exclusion could be sustained. The dominance of the medical profession ensured that even considerable patient support and the support of numerous parliamentarians was insufficient for chiropractic to be legitimated. For this reason there was little reaction from organised medicine to chiropractic in the first decades—it was considered not worthy of being called a threat. Only later in the period to be considered was organised medicine mobilised into active opposition.

Hence the operation of exclusion as a mode of domination within the health system to be examined in this chapter. It was possible because of state patronage of medicine which allowed medicine to exclude chiropractic as a competitor for its occupational territory. A precondition for the operation of exclusion it should be noted is its situation in a capitalist society. Knowledge is a form of private property under capitalism reflected in laws such as copyright, patents and registration, and to be used for private gain (despite the service ethic) by the possessors of that knowledge. In this respect of course, chiropractors are really no different; their attempt to gain legitimacy is basically a struggle to improve their share of these rewards.

The origins of chiropractic

Chiropractic originated from the United States at the end of the nineteenth century. Its origins in both the United States and later in Australia were connected with the emergence of another alternative mode, that of osteopathy. Both use manipulation of the patient by the practitioner as their principal therapeutic technique. Therapeutic manipulation as a form of healing however has been practised for centuries. Practitioners of manipulation, at least in the Western world, came to be known as bonesetters. As Inglis (1964: 94) argues: 'Since humans began to walk on two legs they have always been particularly susceptible to strains, sprains and dislocations and in time individuals emerged who happened to have the knack of putting things to rights again—a knack which in time developed into a craft handed down from father to son.' From the start in Britain, Inglis argues, bonesetting was part of unorthodoxy, being regarded more as a knack than a craft, although some well known and successful bonesetters emerged. By the end of the nineteenth century bonesetters flourished all over Britain. Bonesetters also were flourishing in the United States by the mid-nineteenth century as Lomax (1975: 11–15) documents. Some of the ideas subsequently incorporated into chiropractic were also found at the time, even amongst medical orthodoxy.

The concept of 'spinal irritation' for instance emerged as a new clinical entity, part of the plethora of theories of disease found in the early nineteenth century. It embraced a variety of nervous symptoms and became a fashionable diagnosis, the key symptom being tenderness on pressure over the vertebral spines. Both chiropractic and osteopathy Lomax (1975: 15) argues were legitimate offsprings of contemporary medical thought.

Osteopathy was developed by Andrew Taylor Still, an allopathic medical practitioner from rural Virginia who became disillusioned with orthodox medicine of the day. Still focussed on the structure of the body, believing structural soundness to be essential to proper functioning. Structural disturbances (strains, slips, dislocations, malpositions of bones) he believed could be adjusted and rectified by manipulation. Once sound, the body's own life force could assert itself to ensure proper functioning and restore health (Inglis, 1964: 99). Still began practising osteopathy in 1874 and in 1892 set up a school to train others at Kirkville, Missouri. Osteopathy developed alongside chiropractic and flourished. In the United States the differences between osteopathy and orthodox medicine gradually narrowed and it eventually became incorporated into medicine. Osteopathy in Australia however developed more from the British context where American trained practitioners went soon after the turn of the century. In Britain and Australia by contrast with the United States, osteopathy has not moved closer to medicine and retains the 'alternative' health status that chiropractic has. The differences between osteopathy and chiropractic are ones of terminology and technique. Chiropractors focus more specifically on the spine while osteopaths stress the interrelationship of all bodily systems. Their more general approach took them closer to medicine, a factor which helps explain their eventual incorporation into orthodox medicine.

The 'discoverer' of chiropractic was Daniel David Palmer who had been a magnetic healer (a form of hypnotherapy) for ten years previous to 1895 when chiropractic was established in Davenport, Iowa. While manipulation had long existed as a therapeutic technique and similar theories of health and illness were found at the time, what Palmer did was to found the occupation of chiropractic. The story of the 'discovery' which has been widely told involved Palmer's janitor who had gone deaf seventeen years previously. Palmer adjusted a vertebra in the janitor's neck and his hearing was restored. Though attested by the janitor's own doctor, the cure was dismissed by doctors as a fluke or scientifically impossible (Gibbons, 1976b: 4). This medical opposition determined Palmer to develop a therapeutic technique based on his discovery. An early patient and associate suggested the name chiropractic from the Greek mean literally 'done by hand'. The theory Palmer developed was, like Still's, that functional disturbance (ill health) was caused by anatomical faults which caused abnormal nerve function. Illness could be treated by manipulating the spine to adjust its anatomical structure so as to remove 'subluxations' or minor spinal displacements. It was these subluxations which caused nerve irritation and eventually illnesses. Thus corrected, the body's life force could restore it to good health. Palmer believed that all disorders originated in the spinal column, not 'caused' by these subluxations as such; rather their existence disturbed the functional balance of the body which could result in disease.

After developing his theory and treatment, Palmer established the Palmer Infirmary and Chiropractic Institute in Davenport, Iowa, in 1897. The early years were marked by a struggle for the survival of chiropractic and Palmer himself spent six months in jail in 1903 for the unlicensed practice of medicine. Differences of opinion as to what constituted chiropractic were present from the start. The first of many splits occurred about 1903 when three of the graduates from the Palmer Infirmary set up the American School of Chiropractice in Cedar Rapids. Palmer's son, BJ Palmer (styled 'the Developer') graduated in 1902 and became involved with the college. Other splits occurred including a bitter one between father and son and DD Palmer the elder sold his equity and moved out to found other schools. He died in 1913, allegedly the result of injuries received when he was hit by an automobile driven by his son (see Gibbons, 1980).

Chiropractors were branded as incompetent quacks or hopeless cultists by orthodox medicine from the start. Yet osteopaths, having a broadly similar theory of disease and treatment, were treated more mildly as irregular and sectarian by orthodox medicine. Osteopathy was seen as one of the many 'irregular' schools of medicine in the United States in the late nineteenth century. According to Wardwell (1978: 9) Still , the founder, conceived of osteopathy as being not in opposition to orthodox medicine but as a means of reforming medicine away from its penchant for large doses of drugs and rudimentary, dangerous surgery. The different reception can be explained to a considerable extent in class terms and is important to the subsequent development of chiropractic. Whereas Still came from a professional family and had been a medical practitioner, Palmer came from a poor rural background having worked in a variety of occupations before discovering chiropractic.

Physicians at the time were themselves struggling for upward social mobility and did not hesitate to stress the humble origins of chiropractic as a way of denigrating it. As Fishbein, long-time spokesman of the American Medical Association, wrote in 1925: 'osteopathy is essentially a method of entering medicine by the back door ... chiropractice by contrast is an attempt to arrive through the cellar.'

For all that, as Gibbons (1976b) argues, histories of chiropractic have tended to underestimate the extent of medical involvement in the establishment of chiropractic. While most of the early students were tradesmen and such, a third of the early graduates from Palmer's institute were medical physicians. Licensed doctors of medicine filled the positions of first editor of his journal, first dean of the school, first clinical director and first chiropractic textbook author. Most of these physician-chiropractors Gibbons argues, were subsequently shunned by the medical world, but not all. Some retained hospital connections and staff appointments elsewhere. One of Palmer's early medical associates, Alvah Gregory (with whom he established a school of chiropractic in Oklahoma City), attempted to justify Palmer's unorthodoxy to the medical world in his 1910 book on *Spinal Adjustment*.

> Some of the medical profession and others of the better educated class of people have felt that because spinal adjustments were first introduced by a man who was wholly uneducated in therapeutic lines, he could not have made any discovery of much consequence or importance as a therapeutic auxiliary but this does not by any means, follow. (Quoted in Gibbons, 1976b: 5)

The response of the medical establishment to this new approach to healing developed by an uneducated upstart was to claim that it was sheer quackery. Certainly the formative period of chiropractic development had cultist overtones. DD Palmer imbued it with an evangelical mystique and even dabbled in the metaphysical attributing the gaining of his chiropractic principles to 'conversations' he claimed to hold with a Davenport physician who died 30 years before Palmer announced his discovery and with whom he had never met. Chiropractic theory became dogma and dissenters were expelled from the ranks. As a result Gibbons (1976b: 10) argues of the United States:

> The history of chiropractic through much of this century has been one of trial and turmoil, schism and sectarianism, dogma and debate. The earliest schools were many times launched after violent disagreements between the Discoverer and the Developer and their followers over the emphasis upon adjusting techniques for particular regions of the spine, over the means of diagnosis and over curriculum.

In understanding the origins of chiropractic however, the social context in which it appeared has to be considered. As medical historians have shown, this was a time of proliferation of medical sects and other equally colourful instances of founding, school proliferation and internal division exist. In the face of medical opposition, Palmer's attitude that chiropractic was the opposite of medicine, hardened. His son BJ Palmer intensified this stance in an aggressive fashion, arguing that chiropractic was 'separate and distinct from medicine', and the pattern of relationship which dominated relations between medicine and chiropractic was set. A vocabularly was developed to express the difference between chiropractic and medicine. Hence chiropractors do not 'treat', they 'adjust' in 'offices', not 'rooms'. They 'analyse' the spine rather than 'diagnose', they study 'symptomatology' rather than 'pathology' and 'roentology' rather than 'radiology'.

In view of the early difficulties, trenchant medical opposition and the failure of many other medical sects, the fact that chiropractic survived at all let alone flourished is itself interesting. Several reasons would appear to account for its survival. First among these, Wardwell (1978) argues, is the vested economic and professional interest of BJ Palmer, which led him to struggle to keep chiropractic separate and distinct. With considerable business skill (extending well beyond the chiropractic college to radio stations and other business enterprises), BJ Palmer built up a successful publishing business, selling to chiropractors millions of pamphlets, magazines and texts extolling the virtues of chiropractic. Without these vested interests in chiropractic, Wardwell (1978: 12) argues, 'BJ Palmer would probably not have been motivated to fight so hard to keep chiropractic separate and distinct from osteopathy, naturopathy and medicine'. And fight hard he did. In the BJ Palmer era there developed the internal division which has affected chiropractic through to the present day. This division is between the 'straights' who followed Palmer's dictum that only adjustment of the spine by the hand constituted chiropractic; as compared with the 'mixers' who combined spinal manipulation with other modalities of treatment such as herbal remedies, homeopathy, colonic irrigation and so on.

The second reason for the survival of chiropractic would appear paradoxically to be medical opposition itself. On one hand considerable public sympathy was aroused towards chiropractors and on the other hand (internal division notwithstanding), it gave them a much greater source of identity, internal solidarity and motivation. As Gibbons (1976a: 7) argues:

It is doubtful if chiropractic would have survived its formative period had the little nucleus of teachers and practitioners around DD Palmer not adhered to genuine belief that they were involved in a threshold science of far reaching importance. The arrest of DD in 1903 and his subsequent conviction and imprisonment for six months for practising medicine without a license was but the beginning of a phase of real persecution and enforced poverty which was to see its full drama played out two decades later when literally hundreds of chiropractors marched to jail in California singing 'Onward Christian Soldiers'.

Yet no healing modality can survive if it cannot attract patients. This aspect of the survival of chiropractic in the United States appears to have been little studied. Some ideas of who the early patients of chiropractors were, and why they attended chiropractors is provided by McCorkle (1961). Based on social anthropological fieldwork in rural Iowa, McCorkle attributes the survival and success of chiropractic in the midwest at least, to its appeal to the rural population of that region, in particular its congruence with rural midwestern belief systems and culture. This congruence was especially amongst the traditional middle class farming population.

> It was founded in the Midwest by a Midwesterner and provides a good fit with several aspects of rural Iowa culture. Rejecting the physicians complicated and not altogether complete theory of the multiple causation of disease, it offers a common sense, single cause theory that is capable of effective presentation by mechanical analogy. The chiropractic system also upholds the sanctity of the human body and makes use of the healing power of the laying on of hands—two things calculated to appeal to people exposed to regular Christian teaching. (McCorkle, 1961: 22)

Chiropractic treatment was seen by the local Iowans as likely to consume less time and cost less money than a medical doctor, 'allowing him to go right back to work' (McCorkle, 1961: 22).

Not only did chiropractic survive, but it began to flourish under the direction of BJ Palmer. A measure of its attractiveness was that from the 1920s it began to attract students from outside America, including Australia, to train as chiropractors, particularly at Palmer College. Having considered the American antecedents, it is now possible to concentrate on the development of chiropractic in Australia. The early development of chiropractic in America is important to its subsequent development in Australia. Faced with opposition from the Australian medical profession, many Australian chiropractors drew their occupational identity and support from the American context.

Chiropractic in Australia

The development of chiropractic in Australia I propose to consider in four periods up until 1978. Like many developing occupations, chiropractic has had its share of 'growing pains'. The major one, which has been important throughout much of its development, has been a division between locally trained and foreign trained practitioners. Those chiropractors who travelled to America or Canada to train regarded themselves as the only ones qualified to be called chiropractors and formed themselves into a separate professional body—the Australian Chiropractors Association (hereafter ACA). The second group were those who received training in chiropractic in Australia, either through an apprentice type training or in a small local college. Without registration anyone could call themselves a chiropractor, whether trained or not. This local faction is associated with the development of osteopathy and eventually formed themselves into a separate professional association, the United Chiropractors Association (hereafter UCA). The existence of these two factions has been a major feature of the development of chiropractic and overshadowed the straights/mixers division which was important in the United States. In each of the periods to be analysed the development of both factions needs to be considered.

The process to be analysed here is the creation of the occupation chiropractic; its establishment and development in the face of staunch medical opposition and its struggle to professionalise and gain social mobility for its members. The process is an interesting one in sociological terms; the establishment of a new occupation aiming to secure a niche in an existing division of labour. What also makes it interesting, in fact probably unique, is that its very existence was challenged and opposed from the outset by a much larger and more powerful occupation, with the benefit of state patronage. The struggle to achieve an occupational territory of its own within a rigid and hierarchical division of labour sheds considerable light on the process of legitimation—of both the occupation itself and the knowledge upon which that occupation is based.

The establishment period, 1918–1953

Prior to 1945 the numbers of chiropractors were very small; those locally trained tended to practise it as one of a number of healing modalities used and only the American trained practitioners really used it exclusively. The impact of chiropractic in this era was thus minimal and as such it attracted little attention from medicine. Most of medicine's attention in this early period was directed at the controlling of homeopathy, which was the major competitor and most popular 'alternative' healing modality at the time. In a previous chapter the process of controlling homeopathy through the 1908 Medical Registration Act was analysed. Chiropractic in this era had not stood out as a threat to medical dominance and constituted just one of a number of healing modalities which existed outside orthodox medicine.

a) *The Locals*: The locally trained group of chiropractic practitioners in Victoria evolved from the practice of osteopathy, derived not so much directly from the United States but indirectly via Great Britain. As Campbell (1980) points out, British osteopathy was somewhat different from the American mode and placed greater emphasis on natural therapies than medical ones. In other words it was more oppositional from the outset than in America. This, and a much more firmly entrenched medical profession in Britain, meant that osteopathy has remained an 'alternative' mode in Great Britain and Australia and has not been incorporated into medicine as it has in the United States.

The practice of osteopathy in Victoria began in the first decade of the twentieth century. The dominant figure in this strand of the development of chiropractic was FG Roberts who was first and foremost an entrepreneur with many business ventures including rest homes and a chain of health food stores. Roberts himself practised variously as a herbalist, naturopath and osteopath. He set up clinics all around Australia and visited these regularly. Although beyond the period currently under consideration, it is worth noting Roberts' subsequent activities. He took a leading role in the United Practitioners Association and also established the British and Australian Institute of Naturopathy to train practitioners in the healing arts. In 1959 this became the Chiropractic and Osteopathy College of Australasia. Roberts appears to have never visited the United States although he did receive the curricula and teaching manuals from two chiropractic colleges there. The Victorian Committee of Inquiry into Osteopathy, Chiropractic and Naturopathy (hereafter the Ward Report, 1975: 6), concluded, 'FG Roberts was obviously a man with a flair for adopting fashions in the healing arts and consequently had little difficulty in using various methods of healing which captured the imagination of supporters of drugless therapies in various forms for more than fifty years'.

b) *The Foreigners*: The other faction in the development of chiropractic in Australia was those practitioners who had received their training in the United States, principally at Palmer College, and began to practise in Australia from about the end of the First World War. Several of this early group were New Zealanders. Cecil Wells for instance went to Palmer College from New Zealand, graduating in 1926. He practised in Hobart for seven years before arriving in Melbourne in 1933. Wells bought the practice from a chiropractor named Smiley who appears to have been the first trained chiropractor in Victoria, having begun to practise about the time of the first world war. The numbers grew slowly so that by 1938 there were still less than ten American trained practitioners. This group would have nothing to do either professionally or socially with the local 'untrained' chiropractors, regarding them as 'quacks'. Of course the cost of receiving American training in chiropractic severely limited the numbers able to go. Cecil Wells for instance was able to go on an inheritance received from his family.

Others went on a shoestring budget. One such early chiropractor, now legendary, was 'Macky' Searby who travelled steerage by boat to Los Angeles in the 1920s, then with his pregnant wife pushed a hand-cart with their possessions across the United States to Davenport, Iowa. BJ Palmer made great publicity out of the trip and the cart is now held in the Palmer museum. In fact Searby, a rugged individualist by all accounts, only stayed six months, figuring he had learnt all they could teach him by then, and left without graduating to return to Australia to take up practice. He later received great publicity when he successfully adjusted an injured orang-utan in the Sydney zoo.

During this period the first attempts were made at organising an occupational association, at first with limited success. Then in 1938 the Australian Chiropractor's Association (ACA) was formed at a meeting in Sydney with the aims of improving the status of chiropractic and assisting others to go to America for training. In 1941 the Chiropractors Association of Victoria (CAV) was formed when most foreign-trained Victorian chiropractors split from the ACA, apparently dissatisfied with the domination of the ACA by New South Wales and as a result of a disagreement over the qualifications of a Victorian member. Victoria remained separate until 1961 when it again became the Victorian branch of the ACA.

The first indication which could be found of any concern on the part of medicine towards chiropractic was in 1922 when the executive of the BMA (Victorian Branch) directed its secretary (Dr C Stanton Crouch) to write to the American Medical Association asking for information on 'certain classes of persons who style themselves physiotherapists, mechano-therapists, chiropractors, osteopaths, naturopaths, naprapaths etc'. The letter continued 'this state is fast becoming invaded with a number of persons professedly skilled in the art of healing' (AMA Archives). By the 1930s it appears that chiropractic and osteopathy were beginning to emerge more seriously as more important amongst the range of alternative modalities. An address in 1931 to the Royal Victorian Trained Nurses Association by Alfred J Trinca (1931: 10), a senior surgeon, claimed:

> I will not weary you with details of the methods of the many other forms of Faith healing and exploitation of a sick or imaginary sick public except to state that most of them are offshoots of the parent cults of Osteopathy and Chiropractic. Let us dismiss them with a mere mention of their fantastic appellations—Physiotherapy, mechanotherapy, naturopathy, neuropathy, naprapathy, before I myself am accused of being an adherent of nauseopathy.

The class attitude of the medical profession towards alternative practitioners and their patients, one of arrogant incredulity, is expressed later in the address. 'There is a certain class of mind not very profound or well balanced which is attracted to a new cure by its very novelty and challenge to familiar ways ... The tolerance of these pariahs in our midst is one of the most amazing inconsistencies of our present civilisation.' (Trinca, 1931: 10–11) At the same time the writer castigated fellow members of the medical profession for their inactivity.

Certainly in the period under consideration there is little evidence that chiropractic was considered much of a threat to medicine. Professor Rod Andrew, who graduated in medicine in 1935, recalled

We knew of osteopaths in the community and nobody except the patients who went to them in the medical profession took them seriously. In other words they were not even——, they couldn't have been honoured by being called a threat ... Neither then nor as a student did we ever consider them a threat—it was all part of black magic, sort of chinese herbalist stuff.

The newly formed National Health and Medical Research Council considered chiropractic in its second session in 1937. In evidence it considered a Canadian report done in 1917 when chiropractic had only existed for twelve years, and evidence given before the Select Committee of the House of Lords (date not given). At this session the council resolved 'In view of these reports and of the fact that the Medical Acts of the several states do not recognise chiropraxis, the Council does not consider that there is any reason for further inquiry into the value of the work of chiropractors' (AMA, 1974: Appendix 7). The 26th session of the council endorsed their earlier resolution in November 1948.

The period of expansion, 1954–1961

During this period the number of chiropractors both locally and foreign trained increased considerably. It was also during this period that chiropractors began to seek legitimation for themselves through statutory recognition and access to advantages such as insurance rebates on their fees. Medical opposition in this period remained low key and behind the scenes, medicine relying on the authority of its expertise in the health arena to prevent any recognition of chiropractic. In this period chiropractic emerged as a distinct occupation and strategies for professionalisation were pursued.

a) *The Locals*: As we have seen, FG Roberts continued to be the major figure during this period. More emphasis gradually came to be placed upon chiropractic and osteopathy from amongst the variety of alternative modalities. The first local training institution was the PAX College at Ballarat in the late 1940s, and this together with the Chiropractic and Osteopathic College of Australasia established by Roberts, appears to have trained considerable numbers of chiropractors on a part-time basis (see Webb Report, 1977: 272).

b) *The Foreign-Trained*: From the end of the Second World War American trained chiropractors began to much more actively pursue the professionalisation and legitimation of chiropractic. The CAV, set about substantially increasing the numbers of practitioners of chiropractic. To be established on a more solid footing it was argued, needed much greater numbers in practice. An active recruitment policy was instituted to encourage young Victorians to go to the United States to train. A new period of expansion began in 1954 when a student trust fund was established to assist this process by providing interest-free loans etc. The number of foreign-trained chiropractors increased as a result from seven in 1949 to about 40 in 1960.

During this period also the CAV began to pursue legislation to provide for the registration of foreign-trained chiropractors (only). In this it was spurred on by legislative developments in other states, in particular the exemption of chiropractors from the Medical Practitioners' Act of Western Australia (the first of any sort of statutory recognition of chiropractors). In South Australia the passing of the Physiotherapists' Act of 1945 threatened to outlaw the practice of chiropractic in that state. (The existing practitioners were eligible for registration under a 'grandfather' clause.) Chiropractors were exempted from the act in 1949, following a concerted four year campaign by chiropractors and their patients. Exemptions for chiropractors were gained from various medical and physiotherapy acts in other states including Western Australia in 1951, and New South Wales in 1956 and 1958. In all three cases, political pressure from chiropractors and their growing numbers of patients seems to have been sufficient to result in exemption being granted.

On three occasions during the 1950s deputations were made to the government arguing that registration should be given to chiropractors and only foreign-trained ones at that. Statutory recognition, they argued, would lead to recognition by workers' compensation boards and insurance companies (resulting in a saving to the economy of the country) and allow chiropractic patients the right to claim tax deductions on their treatment as they would with treatment by doctors. The CAV in their journal *Chiropractic* (Jan., 1959: 10) was quite open about their aim to 'wipe out the unqualified practitioner' and 'prevent unscrupulous people from advertising that they could teach chiropractic in Victoria without adequate facilities or qualifications'. The latter meant of course, the Roberts School. The CAV gave evidence before a parliamentary subcommittee set up to examine the issue in 1959. However the government's decision was that it did not intend to proceed with legislation 'at this stage' (Chiropractic, Jan., 1959: 3). Other strategies in the attempt to secure registration included wining and dining of politicians, holding public meetings and attempting to mobilise patient support for chiropractic.

None of these strategies bore fruit however. A confidential AMA document of 1966 reveals that pressure was brought to bear on the parliamentary parties and this would appear to be the reason why the chiropractors' attempts to secure registration were unsuccessful.

> ... It is necessary that no occasion to influence the views of individual members of Parliament should be lost, and this was done most successfully in 1958 when a document entitled 'What is Chiropractic?' was prepared by Dr CH Dickson and circulated to selected members of the Victorian Branch of the British Medical Association who in turn approached their parliamentary representatives. (AMA, 1966)

Chiropractic's emergence and increasing numbers of practitioners and patients during this period, of course began to affect the attitude of orthodox medicine towards it. At the official level it appears there was little contact. Medical dominance meant that competitors were not likely to be taken very seriously. However at the level of the individual practitioner it was different. In metropolitan Melbourne chiropractors and doctors could go their own way without much contact. Mrs Fyvie Wells, wife of Cecil Wells, recalls: 'We went steadily on in our own quiet way. We never wanted to draw attention. We felt that chiropractic could stand on its own merit and we just went quietly on from that.' They had friends who were doctors, but their contact was purely social and not professional and they 'agreed to disagree on medical matters'.

In the rural areas however things were different. Anthony Hart, for instance, went to practise in Morwell in 1949, not long after he returned from the United States. He recalled,

> I was regarded by the local medics as being the incarnation of the antichrist, I mean I was less than the dust and worse than Jack-the-Ripper and anyone who had any brains at all would not go within a bull's roar of the place ... I was told to my face by one of the doctors that I should be ridden out of town, tarred and feathered and what have you.

One specific incidence remained vivid in his memory and concerned the local community service club.

> I was nominated very early in the piece for the local Apex club ... and you know what Apexians are like, if you're warm and breathing

and interested they won't let you out of their sights. You don't need any qualification to be an Apexian, so long as you're not a known criminal you're right. Anyhow I was balloted out of the Morwell Apex Club in 1950 by the local chemist, one of the local doctors, and they enlisted the aid of the local butcher. They needed three objections and they got it and this almost created an incident in the Apex organisation cos it's unheard of for someone to be balloted out of the Apex Club, and the fact that it was simply because someone didn't agree with my profession resulted in all sorts of red faces.

In the period of expansion then, the internal divisions within chiropractic began to emerge as an obstacle to the occupation's professionalisation. Foreign-trained chiropractors opposed those locally trained and both groups were opposed by medicine. As in the United States chiropractors drew much of their occupational identity from its oppositional stance to medicine. This strong belief in the benefits of chiropractic treatment was frequently with great personal cost too. Seeking conventional medical treatment was 'like pork in a kosher butcher's shop' and some medical conditions which would probably have benefitted by a visit to a medical doctor, went untreated.

The period of agitation, 1961–1973

During this period agitation for the statutory recognition and registration of chiropractic intensified. The features of the earlier period continued; the split between the locally trained and foreign-trained chiropractors, and the opposition to both by orthodox medicine. In this period a new group emerged to oppose chiropractic as well. The occupational territory claimed by physiotherapy overlapped with that of chiropractic and physiotherapy joined the fray, along with medicine, against chiropractic. This period also sees the first of the many commissions of inquiry into chiropractic, which although held in Western Australia had ramifications that were felt across Australia including Victoria.

The early part of the decade was spent in attempting to gain support from the various political parties. Both the locally trained and foreign-trained associations attempted to do this, the foreign-trained practitioners arguing that they only should be registered while the locals argued that all should be. A committee was set up by the Labor Party to consider chiropractic in 1960 and received representations from interested parties such as both the foreign and locally trained associations, orthodox medicine and physiotherapy. Their report, presented in 1963, was however a rebuff for chiropractic, arguing against statutory recognition (The Age, 10.6.1963). Other political parties including the Democratic Labor Party and the Country Party did support chiropractic registration. In the ruling Liberal Party however while there was some support from individual members, the medical lobby against chiropractic was too strong. A 'Case for defining the status of the Chiropractic Profession' had been put before the Parliamentary Liberal and Country Parties in 1960, but no action resulted. Evidence given before the Ward Inquiry (Transcripts, 1969: 298) revealed that again in 1969, representatives of the AMA had argued to the health and social services committee of the Liberal Party that chiropractors and osteopaths were in many instances a menace to health. Professor Rod Andrew summed up medical opposition to chiropractic, an element of which appears to have been class opposition.

> If you're in the Church of Spain you're not awfully keen on Seventh Day Adventists—you tend to keep those funny people out and the same in medicine with its monopoly ... They naturally wanted to keep them out, they hadn't had a proper education, they weren't gentlemen, their intellectual base to say nothing of their scientific base hardly existed and up till ten or fifteen years ago, they were the most extraordinarily diverse kind.

In an attempt to gain support for chiropractic registration, the foreign-trained practitioners concentrated their efforts on those segments of the population which were likely to suffer from the sort of musculoskeletal problems which chiropractors claimed to be able to help; that is those with non-sedentary occupations such as the farming community. There seems little doubt that substantial support was forthcoming from this group and chiropractors were able to assist in back problems incurred in farming life. Country Party support was one measure of this; support was also forthcoming from the Australian Primary Producers Union, the Victorian Dairy Farmers Association, the Victorian Wheat and Wool Growers Association, and the Country Women's Association of Victoria (*Chiropractic*, March, 1963: 25). To gain publicity for chiropractic in 1963, a 'Survey of Spinal Injuries Among Farmers and Rural Workers' was conducted on an Australia-wide basis by the Victorian organisation (*Chiropractic*, Christmas, 1960: 16–17). Another group to support chiropractic, particularly in workers compensation cases, was mining unions such as the Barrier Industrial Council in Broken Hill (*Chiropractic*, Christmas, 1960: 20).

Further major effort continued to be put into attracting more Victorians to train as chiropractors. The journal of the ACA actively encouraged applications from interested persons for loans from the student Trust Fund to enable travel to the United States for training. In 1963 overseas scholarships were established at some chiropractic colleges in the United States and Canada for Australian students endorsed by the ACA. These provided exemption from fees charged by the colleges and were utilised to maximum advantage.

From 1960 also the foreign-trained chiropractors at least, began to get their own house in order. A study of chiropractic around Australia was carried out by Mr AW Rogers, the solicitor for the CAV. His recommendation was for a national association with state autonomy. As a result one of the divisions within the occupation was healed in 1961 with the CAV becoming the Victorian Branch of the Australian Chiropractors Association. With greater unity, at least amongst foreign-trained practitioners, a more active and militant policy of professionalisation could be followed. The code of ethics which the CAV had had all along was tightened and several practitioners who were considered to be using misleading advertising were expelled from the ACA. Those expelled formed another splinter group, the Victorian Society of Chiropractors.

Amongst the locally trained chiropractors there was considerable upheaval in the early 1960s at the end of the FG Roberts era. This appears to have occurred along a straights/mixers dimension. Those who chose to become chiropractors primarily, with very limited or no use of other modalities, broke away to form the United Chiropractors Association (ie chose to throw their lot in with chiropractic). The mixers on the other hand, who saw themselves as applying a variety of modalities of treatment, one of which was chiropractic, formed the Australian Chiropractors', Osteopaths' and Naturopathic Physicians' Association Limited (ACONPAL).

The beginning of this period also saw the first of many official commissions of inquiry into chiropractic in Australia. Pressure from chiropractors in Western Australia and considerable support from the leader of the Western Australian parliamentary opposition, Tonkin, led to the establishment of a committee of inquiry to consider 'fringe' medical modalities. This became a Royal Commission in 1960 and its report was very supportive of chiropractic. In particular it set the pattern for the differential treatment of chiropractic to other 'alternative' modes such as naturopathy and homeopathy. The report recommended that chiropractors (and not the others) be registered and that a 'grandfather' clause allow Australian-trained practitioners registration if they had been in practice five years or more. In considering training facilities the committee inspected the Chiropractic and Osteopathic College of Australasia in Melbourne, the local training institution, but considered it unsatisfactory as it did other training institutions in Australia, and recommended American training as the best available (the Guthrie Report, 1961). In 1964 the Western Australia Chiropractors' Act was passed, accepting the recommendations of the commission, thus making Western Australia the first state to

accord statutory recognition to chiropractors. Chiropractors furthermore constituted a majority on the registration board.

But the hopes of Victorian chiropractors, that Western Australia
would set the precedent for Victoria to follow, were dashed. The
effect of the passing of the Western Australian bill was to harden
medical opposition considerably and make it much more overt than it
had previously been. Suddenly chiropractic had to be taken seriously
as a threat and the Australian Medical Association reacted strongly
where previously most of the activity had been behind the scenes. An
AMA document of 1966 argued: 'The medical profession in Victoria
has been fortunate in having two successive Ministers of Health whose
uncompromising opposition to chiropractic claims has been in large
part responsible for their failure to so far attain their objective.'

Faced with the chiropractors, the Fourth Federal Assembly resolved
that 'The Australian Medical Association is of the opinion that
medical practitioners may not act in consultation with, associate professionally with, conduct investigations for, or refer patients to chiropractors and osteopaths' (AMA, 1966).

This ethical injunction was backed with the power of deregistration
for doctors who contravened it, through the influence of the AMA
over the Medical Board of Victoria. Whatever individual doctors may
have thought of chiropractors, the complete autonomy to manage its
own internal affairs granted through the Medical Board in the Medical
Act of 1933 meant that it could be enforced (MJA Supplement,
19.6.1965: 127). There is some evidence of the AMA being willing to
take this extreme step. As one chiropractor recalled,

> In the mid-sixties several chiropractors got to know that a certain
> diagnostician in St Kilda Road was willing to take referrals from
> chiropractors and give a report back and so we started sending
> tricky cases on to him, and that was lovely for about a year and then
> the AMA got wind of it and threatened him with expulsion and he
> had to refuse.

In opposing the registration of chiropractors the AMA saw itself as
acting in the public interest, as an editorial (MJA, 26.11.1966: 1047)
claimed: 'The obligation to educate and inform the uninformed or
gullible about cults and their practitioners is as much the business of
doctors as to vaccinate those exposed to smallpox.'

In the same article the AMA demonstrated a sensitivity to the claim
that it was attempting to monopolise the health field:

> ... one of the dangers of present attempts by the chiropractors to
> gain official recognition is that those with legislative authority,
> anxious to keep democracy afloat, may be mislead into believing
> that opposition by the medical establishment is equivalent to the

powerful majority striving to gag the faint voiced minority, a state of affairs not to be tolerated. (MJA, 26.11.1966: 1047)

The concern at the possibility of chiropractic registration in Victoria was expressed in the 1966 background paper on chiropractic written by the medical secretary of the AMA. It drew mainly on American material to evaluate chiropractic, in particular that provided by the American Medical Association's Department of Investigation, though it did also utilise a pseudo-patient. The report found there were powerful forces working towards registration in Victoria. These included increasingly militant occupational associations able to mobilise considerable patient support, as well as support from other groups such as primary producer organisations and some minor political parties. Chiropractic in other words was drawing on its clinical legitimacy (ie with patients) to press for politico-legal legitimacy. The AMA advised against any form of registration.

The Government of Victoria has the responsibility of ensuring that the highest standards of health and medical care are maintained in this community. This idea cannot be reconciled with the idea of affording legal status and recognition to the followers of a pseudo-medical cult completely lacking any scientific basis. It is the continuing obligation of the medical profession to be active in opposition to any such ill-advised proposal. (AMA, 1966: 16)

In 1966 the AMA was invited by the state government to investigate chiropractic and report on the advisability of statutory registration. A science subcommittee was set up and its report of 1967, accepted by the AMA, not surprisingly advised against registration. However it did set down minimum criteria under which registration should be considered. These included accreditation of chiropractic training schools by a recognised educational or academic institution, with registration restricted to graduates of those schools only, and educational training 'nothing less than what is required of other paramedical bodies' (Andrew, 1979: 2).

The intention of the committee and the AMA was clear, as Professor Rod Andrew, a member of the committee recalls, 'The AMA committee at the time thought they'd built enough walls and dug a deep enough ditch and filled that with enough bullshit to make it impossible for any chiropractic group ever to fulfill all those conditions'.

The AMA communicated their report to the state government but apparently not to the chiropractors themselves who eventually learnt of the minimum criteria three and a half years later, when they requested discussions with the AMA in 1971 in an attempt to establish better relations. The ACA responded with an analysis of the AMA paper given to the state Minister of Health in which they challenged some statements of fact but basically agreed with the criteria set out, claiming American and Canadian chiropractic schools provided adequate training in the areas the AMA specified (ACA, 1971). Since there was little disagreement the ACA argued legislation could proceed.

In fact it was becoming widely recognised by this time that the major need for chiropractic was an acceptable Australian training institution. As the AMA paper pointed out, no American degree had any official standing in Australia, and to recognise chiropractic qualifications would be setting a major precedent. Both factions of chiropractors were by this time aware of this need. The locals had set up their own training institution but without any official encouragement or the support of the foreign-trained practioners could not raise it to a sufficient standing to be acceptable. Staff with academic qualifications could not be attracted, especially in the basic biomedical sciences and courses were often taught by medical students. In 1964, FG Roberts led a deputation of locals to see the then minister of health seeking registration, but was advised that a training institution of acceptable standards would have to be established before registration could be considered. Following this deputation, the Chiropractic and Osteopathic College of Australasia was incorporated and later renamed the Chiropractic College of Australasia (the Ward Report, 1975: 6).

The ACA had also been conscious for many years of the need for an Australian training institution of acceptable standards. However the small number of chiropractors in Australia was a considerable impediment to the establishment of an acceptable training course because of the high cost involved. With little hope of gaining entry into the established tertiary education system, the foreign-trained chiropractors were faced with setting up their own institution. As the secretary of the association wrote in 1960,

> We realise that to have proper legal standing we will have to establish a chiropractic school approved by law but before we open a school we will need some official encouragement ... For every Victorian student now in the United States there must be nine or ten who want to go there but cannot because of cost of family commitments. (Chiropractic, Dec., 1969: 13)

Even in 1960 there was support for training at the Royal Melbourne Institute of Technology (RMIT) through its principal Mr R Mackay, a longtime chiropractic patient; support which was to bear fruit in the 1970s. In 1972 the Joint Australasian Committee on Chiropractic Education was established by the ACA and the New Zealand Chiropractors' Association to establish a chiropractic training course in Australasia.

By the 1960s also physiotherapy had dropped its 'fringe' medicine tag through accepting subordination to medical dominance in agreeing to treat only on referral from a medical practitioner. The occupational territory claimed by chiropractors conflicted not only with the medical profession by claiming to provide a complete alternative system of health care, but also with physiotherapy in claiming special expertise in musculoskeletal disorders, those that physiotherapists also claimed to be able to treat. Through the 1960s, it appears, the physiotherapists became increasingly concerned about the 'threat of chiropractors'. A meeting of interested members of the Australian Physiotherapists Association in 1967, called to discuss the 'threat to our profession', was addressed by an orthopaedic surgeon who outlined the competition with chiropractors very candidly, telling the meeting 'that physiotherapists' incomes would drop by half if we do not take steps to advance our cause before unlicensed practitioners become registered'. A physiotherapist responded that

> unfortunately in Victoria physios are just not doing their best because of a lack of knowledge and training in manipulation whereas the opposition are far more skilled operators. However through post graduate lectures and courses, and localised meetings, we can outstrip the others because of our basic medical knowledge and our contacts in the medical field. However let us remember that the *enemy* can teach us a lot and we should not be slow to take advantage of this. (Quoted in ACA, 1974a: 50–54; emphasis added)

The meeting resolved to suggest the formation of an association of manipulative therapists to the APA, and advocated the expansion of the occupational territory of physiotherapy to include manipulation.

Towards the end of 1972 the debate to come to a head. The ACA offered to hold talks with the AMA, offering to relinquish to medical specialists the taking of X-rays as a carrot. Then on 18 December the Victorian cabinet gave the approval for parliamentary draftsmen to begin preparing a registration bill (VPD, 338, 1978: 3253). A newspaper report on 22 February 1973 under the heading 'Quackery to be eliminated' announced that draft legislation to register chiropractors would be going before parliament the next week (The Age, 22.2.1973). In the meantime however, anti-chiropractic forces swung into action. The *Herald* of the same day announced that the AMA 'wants to meet the Premier to protest against the proposed bill to register chiropractors' (The Herald, 22.2.1973). The report quoted the secretary of the AMA as indicating that the government had promised to consult it before drafting any legislation registering chiropractors. An AMA paper entitled 'Chiropractic 1973' was circulated to all parliamentarians. The Australian Physiotherapy Association also made submissions to the Victorian government, opposing registration (APA, 1973). In a section entitled 'The Encroachment of Chiropractic on the Realms of Physiotherapy' the submission argued,

... Whilst admitting the value of these procedures (eg electro-therapy and traction) as an aid to spinal treatment, we abhor chiropractors stealing our treatment methods and lobbying to be registered as a separate profession.
Whilst we acknowledge the benefits of manipulation in appro-priately selected cases, we resent the chiropractors extracting this one aspect of our treatment and endeavouring to obtain registration as a rival profession. (APA, 1973: 3)

The opposition of the AMA and the physiotherapists would appear to have changed the government's mind. A letter from the federal executive of the AMA to all branches, dated 26 March 1973, gave a report of the meeting with the Premier of Victoria, Mr Hamer, indicating that they had been given a 'firm assurance that legislation to register chiropractors has been abandoned, and that an all party enquiry would be held if the Liberal Party was re-elected in the forth-coming state elections'. The report concluded 'we were very satisfied with the results of the meeting with the Premier' (ACA Archives). A deputation from the ACA was advised later in 1973 by the Premier that registration would not be effected in Victoria until a tertiary level course had been established in Victoria, indicating that he 'was not prepared to have a profession available only to people able to afford the high expense of overseas education ("an elitist group")' (PIT, 1978).

So the period of agitation in the development of chiropractic ended without success in achieving statutory registration and recognition. Internal disunity and opposition from orthodox medicine and physio-therapy would appear to explain this. Medical dominance ensured that even considerable patient support and the support of a number of parliamentarians was insufficient to achieve politico-legal legitimacy. In this period however chiropractic made considerable progress. The number of practitioners for instance increased enormously, from probably something less than 50 chiropractors in various organisa-tions in various organisations in 1960 to about 180 in 1973 (the Ward Report, 1975: 9). Another significant advance made during this period was the extension of health insurance cover to include chiropractic consultation. This development reflected the growing clinical legiti-macy of chiropractic. The Australian Natives Association was the first to offer rebates in the early 1960s, along with several smaller funds. Others extended their cover in waves, a sort of domino effect, another one being in the late 1960s when Manchester Unity extended its cover. The last to 'fall' was the Medical Benefits Fund in 1980, historically closely aligned with the AMA. Rebates were claimable from both local and foreign-trained chiropractors.

The other important development in this period was a change in the level of discourse at which the struggle was conducted. Prior to the Guthrie Inquiry in Western Australia the discourse had been mainly at the level of rhetoric. With the establishment of committees of inquiry which became increasingly important, the rhetoric gave way to reasoned argument as legal counsel became involved on both sides of the struggle.

The period of legitimation, 1973–1978

In this last period under consideration events moved rapidly. As the Victorian Premier had promised in his meeting with the AMA, a committee of inquiry into chiropractic, osteopathy and naturopathy was established in 1973 under the chairmanship of the Hon HR Ward, MLC, following the re-election of the ruling Liberal government. This committee took until late 1975 to produce its report, but it represented the first serious attempt to Victoria to evaluate alternative modes of health care. Interested parties presented submissions which revealed the extent of divisions both within chiropractic and also between chiropractic and orthodox medicine.

A good example of these divisions concerned the taking of X-rays as a diagnostic tool, common to both orthodox medicine and chiropractic. This is a procedure which exposes a patient to a dose of radiation and as such should be minimised. Evidence was given to the enquiry that not only were AMA members refusing to release X-rays to chiropractors when patients transferred, but also the ACA members were refusing to release them to UCA members (considering them 'unqualified'), thereby on each occasion necessitating further X-rays to be taken. Indeed the refusal of an ACA chiropractor to release X-rays to a locally trained one resulted in legal action to secure them, such was the division within chiropractic. The policy of the ACA was to release X-ray photographs only to 'allied' practitioners and locally trained practitioners did not qualify as 'allied'. The submission of the Chiropractic College of Australia (affiliated with UCA), for its part, included a research paper which was critical of the educational qualifications of the faculty of American chiropractic schools, thus undermining the argument of the ACA that only its training was of a sufficient standard to warrant registration. The report found for instance that more than half of the faculties did not have 'recognised' four year academic degrees. Both the AMA and APA submissions were adamantly opposed to any form of registration for either group of chiropractors.

The report of the Ward Committee (1975) however did come out in favour of the registration of chiropractors and osteopaths but in a restricted form, on a restricted occupational territory. Two forms of registration were recommended: 'O' registration which would enable primary contact (ie without medical referral), and 'R' registration which would permit treatment only on written referral by a registered medical practitioner. The report came out strongly against a 'grandfather' clause to allow those already in practice but with doubtful qualifications, to continue practising. On the question of the occupational territory of chiropractors, the committee recommended that chiropractors and osteopaths be restricted to neuro-musculoskeletal disorders rather than being able to treat a range of organic or visceral disorders as well. In other words the claim of chiropractic to be a complete alternative system of health care and thus a direct competitor with the medical profession was rejected. Instead the recommendation was for chiropractors to be given a much more limited occupational territory, and one which brought them more directly into competition with that claimed by physiotherapy. In line with this, the committee recommended unifying the practice of manipulative theraphy under one administration, the Manipulative Therapy Board, with one division dealing with the registration of chiropractors and osteopaths, and the other with physiotherapists and masseurs.

In any registration Act a crucial issue is the composition of the registration board, that is, those who decide who can be registered and who can not. The issue is whether the occupation for whom it is set up has a majority of members on the board and is thus able to control the registration process, or whether they constitute a minority and control is vested outside the occupation. As we have seen, a crucial feature of medical dominance in the health division of labour is that while some occupations exist outside the direct control of the medical profession, indirect control can nonetheless be effected by representation of members of the medical profession on registration boards. In the Ward Report then, it is significant that a majority of chiropractors and osteopaths was *not* recommended for the Chiropractors' and Osteopaths' division of the Manipulative Therapists' Board. Of the seven members, it was recommended that three be from chiropractic and osteopathy (two chiropractors and one osteopath), three from the medical profession (one orthopaedic surgeon, one medical educator and one general practitioner), the seventh position to be held by an academic not involved in teaching medicine (the Ward Report, 1975: 23).

As the Western Australian enquiry had done, the Ward Report also recommended differentiating between chiropractors and osteopaths on one hand, for whom registration was recommended; and other fringe practitioners (in particular naturopaths) on the other, for whom it was not. The report was also critical of the medical opposition to 'fringe' practitioners, arguing that 'the AMA was somewhat inflexible in its views but its contempt did not seem to be based on familiarity' (the Ward Report, 1975: 2). The committee recommended that the AMA's code of ethics be changed to allow for referral of patients to osteopaths and chiropractors.

Following tabling of the report the interested parties were invited to respond. The AMA was scathing in its criticism of the report, calling it 'poor in the quality of its language, format and reasoning', and expressed its anger at the proposal that it 'lower its ethical standards at the whim of the committee' to allow referral. It concluded, 'The Australian Medical Association objects to the whole tenor of the report and will continue to oppose the registration of osteopaths, chiropractors and naturopaths until it is satisfied that these practitioners have had adequate training' (AMA, 1976: 3).

The Victorian Branch of the ACA (1976) issues a 'rebuttal' to the report. While obviously pleased that registration had been recommended, the ACA objected to some of the recommendation. Its main objection was to the proposed Manipulative Therapy Board, thus tying chiropractic in with physiotherapy to a considerable extent and thereby removing some of its separate occupational identity. It also found the lack of a chiropractic majority on the registration board 'completely unacceptable to the profession' (ACA, 1976: 11), suggesting instead a composition of five chiropractors and only two non-chiropractors. Secondly it argued that the report provided an unsatisfactory solution to the problem of the inadequately trained practitioner with the two-pronged strategy of an 'R' registration and no 'grandfather' clause. Given the AMA's opposition to chiropractic, the ACA argued it would be unlikely that 'R' registrants would get enough referrals to survive.

Thirdly, it objected to proposed limitations on the scope of chiropractic practice to neuro-musculoskeletal conditions. It argued in defence of the primary contact status and right to treat visceral or organic conditions that given the established lack of training in manipulation for doctors of medicine, chiropractors were in the best position to 'recognise those conditions which are amenable to chiropractic care and to refer patients to other practitioners when the problem is outside the scope of chiropractic' (ACA, 1976: 5). In all the ACA argued, obviously concerned that the recommendations of the committee might be enacted: 'Were the government and eventually the Parliament of Victoria to act upon the committee's findings without further revision or discussion with the chiropractic profession, a grave injustice would be done to the consumers of the services provided by chiropractors.' (ACA, 1976: 2)

Before the Ward committee had completed its deliberations in Victoria, another committee of inquiry was established into 'alternative' medicine, this time on a federal basis. Under the chairmanship of Professor Edwin Webb, the committee was appointed in 1974 in the latter part of the Whitlam Labor period of government. What was distinctive about this commission was that it went much further in attempting to evaluate chiropractic than previous inquiries had done. It commissioned two pieces of research into chiropractic, one a clinical trial over the treatment of migraines (Parker and Tupling, 1977a, 1977b), the other a sociological study into the utilisation of chiropractic services (Boven et al., 1977a, 1977b, 1977c; Siskind et al., 1977). It also got the various parties together for a seminar on manipulative therapy.

The report of the Webb committee, presented in 1977, advocated registration of chiropractors and osteopaths (under a manipulative therapists' registration act), but not naturopaths or homeopaths. It also strongly advocated the need for uniform legislation throughout the Commonwealth. Like the Ward Report it rejected the claim of chiropractic and osteopathy to being an alternative health system, seeing them instead as specialists in spinal manipulation (the Webb Report, 1977: 103). Once again the chiropractors objected to being designated manipulative therapists, sticking to their occupational identity as chiropractors to differentiate them on one hand from orthodox manipulators (a section of the medical profession and physiotherapy), and on the other from proponents of natural therapies such as naturopathy.

In the meantime however, chiropractic in Victoria had taken seriously the recommendation of the Premier arising from their meeting with him in 1973. In 1974, the ACA produced a draft registration bill which provided registration for graduates of colleges of chiropractic acceptable to the board (comprised of ACA members). A 'grandfather' clause was proposed which would have allowed registration for locally trained chiropractors on fulfillment of fairly stringent conditions. These include at least five years practice, passing an examination, and most importantly having 'used as his description the word "chiropractor".*exclusively* in describing his profession' (ACA, 1974b: 11, emphasis added). The last point is important in achieving 'closure' in the occupation and shutting out the 'mixers' from registration.

In 1974 feasibility studies for establishing a training course with a tertiary institution were prepared by the ACA and the International Chiropractic College (hereafter ICC) was formed. Informal contacts with officials at the Royal Melbourne Institute of Technology led to negotiations with Technisearch, the commercial arm of RMIT, to provide instruction in some of the basic science courses. In late 1974 the UCA got wind of developments and requested a meeting with the

ACA, ICC and Technisearch. At that meeting it was agreed that resources should be pooled to support one Australian College—the ICC.

During January 1975 a subcommittee of members of the ACA and UCA met to thrash out the conditions for a merger of the two associations, the closing down of the Chiropractic College of Australasia (and provision for its students to join the ICC course), and the concerted support for ICC. Negotiations broke down in February however, with rejection by the UCA of ACA conditions for membership. These included provisional membership only for UCA members in the ACA, the practice of chiropractic only, occupational identification as a chiropractor only, and attendance at educational seminars. The UCA rejected the provisional membership condition, the restriction to the practice of chiropractic alone, and the heavy financial commitment towards the ICC which the ACA was insisting on from all practitioners ($1000 each to the college building fund) (the Ward Report, 1975: 79–81).

The ICC began teaching students in association with Technisearch from the beginning of 1975 with 25 students enrolled. The arrangement was not very satisfactory and terminated at the end of 1975. In the meantime however the ICC had negotiated an interim arrangement with the Preston Institute of Technology (PIT) after having had discussions with a number of tertiary institutions including the Lincoln Institute of Health Sciences, the training institution for a number of paramedical occupations including physiotherapy. The PIT/ICC course took its first student intake in 1976 financed partly by the students themselves through fees, but mainly from practising chiropractors who spent $750 000 on the programme between 1976 and 1978.

A bill to register chiropractors was finally introduced and passed in May 1978 after some intense last minute lobbying and some 104 amendments (VPD, 1978). The bill set up the Chiropractors and Osteopaths Registration Board of seven members: three practitioners, three doctors of medicine, and one ministerial nominee. Chiropractors and osteopaths were thus not in the majority despite their argument that they should be. A 'grandfather' clause was inserted allowing registration if the applicant had been in practice for at least three years, and could satisfy the board that he or she 'was professionally competent to practise as a chiropractor or osteopath in Victoria'. The act defined chiropractors' occupational territory primarily as manipulation, but no monopoly on this was given. The act allowed only those registered under the act to sue for fees, but exempted 'where chiropractic and osteopathy is performed or advice given', a large number of occupations including medical practitioners, nurses (under supervision of medical practitioners, registered physiotherapists, chiropractors or osteopaths), chiropodists, registered physiotherapists, and other activities such as face or scalp massage for cosmetic purposes.

The effect of the act however was to drastically alter the position of chiropractic in the health division of labour. From having been excluded throughout its history it moved closer to a position of limitation. Certainly it avoided being subordinated (that is, acting on medical referral). It was not entirely limited furthermore. While recognised as specialising in musculoskeletal disorders, it is important that the occupational territory of chiropractic was not restricted to that alone, and the chiropractor is able to treat some visceral or organic conditions.

But the struggle with orthodox medicine was by no means over. One further development is relevant to our discussion here. Having achieved registration, the question of the siting of the chiropractic training course became crucial as the arrangement with Preston was a purely interim one. An accreditation committee from the Victorian Institute of Colleges (VIC) examined the PIT/ICC course to determine whether it would accept it within the VIC framework. The committee, comprised mainly of senior medical academics, recommended that training in some areas was in fact *too much*—for example, in radiology where it commented, 'this content appears too high, being in excess of the expectation of study in this field by a medical student' (cited in ACA, 1978: 21).

Finally, once registration looked inevitable there was a submission to the VIC that the chiropractic course be sited at the Lincoln Institute rather than continuing at PIT. This would appear on the face of it to be a last ditch stand on the part of the orthodox opponents of chiropractic to bring it under medical control. The Federal Council of the AMA at its meeting in May 1978, after the passing of the bill, recommended that 'any tertiary institution providing courses of education in manipulative therapy should not use the word 'chiropractic' in the title of these courses' (cited in ACA, 1978: 24). The ACA came out adamantly opposed to the idea, seeing it as a plot to destroy chiropractic. 'Having failed through many years of lobbying to prevent the registration of chiropractors it would now appear that the AMA is intent upon forcing chiropractic into a paramedical role, strictly under the control of organised medicine and physiotherapy.' (ACA, 1978: 21) It threatened to go interstate rather than set up in a hostile setting, and argued for remaining at Preston. This it subsequently achieved.

From its American beginnings in the late ninteenth century and its arrival in Australia in the first decades of the twentieth century the occupation of chiropractic struggled to survive and legitimate itself both clinically and politico-legally. The former was achieved quite early, the latter only finally in 1978 in Victoria. Opposition to chiropractic was intense throughout its history, and when added to the considerable internal divisions makes its survival rather remarkable and certainly of considerable interest sociologically. Faced with a challenge to its dominance of the health division of labour, the medical profession sought to exclude chiropractic from any form of statutory recognition. This it succeeded in doing for 60 years. When registration was achieved however, despite medical opposition, the dominance of medicine was not really challenged. By having their occupational territory statutorily defined as principally musculo-skeletal disorders rather than the whole gamut of ills which earlier chiropractors had claimed, chiropractic moved more to a relationship of limitation, akin to that occupied by dentists, optometrists and others. So chiropractic achieved politico-legal legitimation in a way which really left medical dominance unchallenged, although chiropractors retained their primary contact status and the right to treat some organic illnesses. The transition in the structural location of chiropractic from exclusion to limitation was thus the result not only of imposition but also of negotiation. Faced with the inevitability of politico-legal legitimation of chiropractic, medicine was able to negotiate its contined dominance within the health division of labour.

The legitimation of chiropractic

In this chapter so far, I have traced in some detail the historical process of the emergence of chiropractic; its survival, blossoming and eventual legitimation, even in the face of medical opposition. In this final section I propose to attempt an explanation for the process which occurred.

In the discussion so far, the process of legitimacy has been divided into two aspects, clinical and politico-legal. Also important to the analysis here is scientific legitimacy. As I have shown, the basis of medicine's exclusion of chiropractic has been the claim that a scientific basis for chiropractic treatment had not been established, and therefore that statutory registration should not be granted. Chiropractic theory, it was claimed, was incommensurable with 'scientific medicine'; its claims were unproven. In short, it lacked scientific legitimacy. As a result the question of which theory was best at alleviating ill health was not directly confronted.

Yet chiropractic has always claimed to have a scientific basis and thus the question should be empirically solvable. However for a number of reasons this has not been the case. Firstly there are methodological difficulties in determining the relative merits of different forms of treatment, in particular the necessary reliance on subjective evaluation of 'improvement'. Secondly there has been little research into the spine and such research is complicated and expensive. Several reasons for this lack of research exist. From the chiropractic point of view the emphasis has been on survival for the practitioners, and the associations have utilised most of the limited funds available to pursue political ends of statutory recognition rather than promoting research. Secondly, medical dominance has extended to the dissemination of research funds, and spinal research has not had much priority. To argue as orthodox medicine has done, that chiropractic theory is unproven is true, but somewhat unfair in view of the small amount of research into the spine which has been done. As the chiropractors point out, if the money which orthodox medicine has spent in opposing chiropractic had been spent on researching its fundamentals, a lot more would be known.

A considerable number of clinical trials of chiropractic and other forms of treatment have been carried out, of varying thoroughness and sophistication (Kane et al., 1974; Doran and Newell, 1975; Breen, 1977; Parker et al., 1978; Fisk, 1980). The New Zealand report on chiropractic examines all these in detail. The best that can be said of these is that they are inconclusive. A workshop held in the United States in 1975 on 'The Research Status of Spinal Manipulative Theory', a landmark event widely quoted in the literature, found that 'specific conclusions cannot be derived from the scientific literature for or against either the efficacy of spinal manipulative therapy or the pathophysiologic foundations from which it is derived' (Goldstein, 1975: 6). In other words, what research there has been does not 'prove' that chiropractic treatment works, but neither does it disprove it.

But while it might not be scientifically proven, the fact that it has survived let alone flourished demonstrates that it is 'proven' in the area which counts most, with patients. Evidence of scientific effectiveness there may not be, but there is evidence of clinical effectiveness. Research conducted for the Webb inquiry found 250 000 new patients attending practitioners of alternative health care every year (Boven et al., 1977a: 349). High levels of patient satisfaction have been recorded in many studies of chiropractic treatment (eg Kane et al., 1974: 1336). How is this anomaly explained? The New Zealand report on chiropractic (1979: 44) examined this issue and concluded,

> The fact remains that the various chiropractic theories that have been advanced since chiropractic was first developed are properly to be regarded as no more than attempts to explain how chiropractic gets the results it does ... Indeed it is probably true to say chiropractic is a form of treatment still in search of an explanation for its effectiveness.

As a result the Commission decided that 'the efficacy of treatment becomes the important issue in the inquiry rather than the adequacy or inadequacy of the explanations so far advanced in an attempt to account for its apparent successes' (NZ Report, 1979: 45).

The statutory recognition of chiropractic as a body of knowledge and an occupation based upon it meant its politico-legal legitimation. Yet this has not been based on scientific legitimacy but on clinical legitimacy. In other words, while chiropractic has never been successful in proving the theory of ill health upon which its technique of spinal manipulative therapy is based, it has been remarkably successful in legitimating itself where it counts most, with patients. The fact that chiropractic achieved politico-legal legitimation not on the basis of scientific legitimacy as most health occupations have done, but on the basis of clinical legitimacy, is particularly important.

In this case the claim of the medical opponents that chiropractic is unscientific clearly is an ideological argument which has been used to exclude chiropractic. The New Zealand Report (1979: 45) for example, views the medical profession's opposition to chiropractic 'philosophy' as a red herring. Furthermore, as we have seen in a previous chapter, the argument fails to acknowledge that clinical medicine is *based* upon scientific knowledge but involves other sorts of knowledge as well. In other words while 'scientific medicine' has had difficulty claiming it was more successful than alternative medicine, it has always been able to claim it was more scientific. It has thus been legitimated through science and able to have its theory about illness accepted as *the* theory. The claim that chiropractic is unscientific then serves ideological ends to justify its exclusion (see Willis, 1978a: 17).

How then is the clinical success of chiropractic to be explained? Apart from the obvious answer that spinal manipulative therapy may actually work, a number of other explanations have also been put forward. One of these is that the chiropractor may be more interpersonally skilled in the sense of being more attuned to the total needs of the patient than doctors are. As Kane et al. (1974: 1336) argue, 'The chiropractor does not seem hurried. He uses language patients can understand. He gives them sympathy and he is patient with them. He does not take a superior attitude towards them. In summary it is an egalitarian relationship rather than a superordinate subordinate relationship'.

Class differences would appear to be important here. With working class patients especially, the chiropractor may be better able to communicate than is his more socially distant medical counterpart. Parker and Tupling (1976: 375) in their study of psychosocial aspects of chiropractic treatment found that the majority of patients regarded highly the interpersonal skills and technical competence of chiropractors. There is considerable evidence of the importance of the practitioner-patient relationship in effective healing (Bloom, 1965). Balint (1957) for instance, sees the most important element in all remedies as an emotionally satisfactory relationship between practitioner and patient. Certainly much work remains to be done on the psychosocial aspects of treatment, as suggested by the literature on the placebo effect in treatment and which is frequently neglected in the emphasis upon 'hard' science and medical technology.

Some direct evidence is provided in the survey of chiropractors carried out as part of the Victorian Ward inquiry. The chiropractors were requested to provide details of patient visits, hours worked etc for a seventeen week period in 1973 (the Ward Report, 1975: 81). The survey showed that a group of 'leading' chiropractors spent an average of nine minutes with each patient. Comparable figures for medicine are not easily available, though my own research in New Zealand in 1974, in the course of which several hundred consultations with general practitioners were observed, revealed that the average consultation time was more like five minutes (Willis, 1976).

The clinical success of chiropractic thus appears to be explained to a considerable extent by its relationship to orthodox medicine. As one chiropractor interviewed put it, 'the success of nonmedical alternative care procedures are based not so much, on their excellence but on the failure of medicine to provide the care that people need'. There is recognition of this basis to chiropractic within the occupation itself, and in my opinion this sort of explanation goes a long way in explaining the survival of chiropractic. On the basis of their research into the psychosocial aspects of chiropractic treatment, Parker and Tupling (1976: 61) conclude,

> it may be that chiropractors have successfully combined a physiologically effective therapy with an elaborate healing ritual in such a way that they can help more people by spinal manipulation than would respond to a doctor or physiotherapist performing the same manipulation without the trimmings.

Another suggested explanation for clinical success, also made by a chiropractor, was low expectations: 'The patient naturally doesn't expect a great deal from the chiropractor so when he gets satisfaction or improvement he's of course highly delighted.'

Clinical success however was insufficient to prevent or modify exclusion throughout most of the period considered. Indeed in the first decades there was little overt organised medical opposition. Chiropractic was simply not considered much of a threat. Medical dominance was achieved and sustained through state patronage which ensured the dominance of its authority in all health matters. This dominance extended throughout society, in both government departments and private companies. In 1974 the ACA wrote to the then minister for Repatriation and Compensation (John Wheeldon) requesting that chiropractic be recognised as a form of medical treatment under the Repatriation Act. The minister responded that 'certain serious obstacles preclude the commission's recognition of chiropractors' services'. The most important of these was that,

> Repatriation's treatment scheme is medically oriented, revolving around referral for specialist or ancillary services by a medical practitioner. It is considered that there has not yet been sufficient evidence tendered to warrant departure from the principle of medical referral and while the Australian Medical Association's refusal to officially recognise or to professionally associate with chiropractors continues, there appears to be little possibility of chiropractors being able to participate in the repatriation treatment scheme. (Correspondence, ACA Archives)

In gaining insurance refunds for its patients also, chiropractors ran into medical dominance. In May 1960, a 'prominent Melbourne insurance assessor' explained why few insurance companies would pay claims for chiropractic treatment, saying that 'Payment of claims lodged with insurance companies was largely governed by medical assessment of the case and while the BMA opposed chiropractic it was impossible for companies to pay claims not cleared by their medical sections' (*Chiropractic*, July, 1960: 23).

Sometimes the exclusion operated indirectly by means of a Catch-22 situation. One of the arguments used against chiropractic registration was that their training courses were inferior and inadequate. Yet part of the reason registration was sought was so that educational courses could be upgraded. It was the lack of registration that in fact prevented the improvement of training courses (Willis, 1978a). Likewise the lack of statutory recognition meant insurance firms could not distinguish between genuine or qualified chiropractors, and others.

The process of exclusion

Given the longstanding denial of politico-legal legitimacy to chiropractic then, how is its final achievement to be explained? In view of the arguments outlined above it may have appeared unlikely that chiropractic would ever achieve statutory recognition at all. The reasons for its success in the 1970s therefore need to be considered in this final section. There are a number of factors which explain this, some of which are recognised by the chiropractors themselves—the result of active pursuit by them in their attempts to secure a position within the health division of labour.

The main factor is the growth in the number of practitioners operating in the community. Beginning in the era of expansion there was an active policy, particularly by the ACA component, to recruit prospective chiropractors and materially assist them to go to the United States for training. As a result the numbers of chiropractors increased substantially from the end of the Second World War but particularly during the 1960s. This had two effects. Firstly chiropractic became much more visible and an increasing proportion of the population came in contact with them. This contact then could be mobilised in the form of patient support for political purposes to lobby for registration.

What seems to have made considerable impact on the various commissions of inquiry was the fact that by the 1970s, large numbers of people were visiting chiropractors and the weight of public opinion was considerable. Chiropractic furthermore had stood the test of time. Any healing modality which fails to attract patients cannot survive and many have not. With clinical legitimation the chiropractors kept agitating and lobbying for recognition, and with the 'inevitability of gradualism' as one chiropractor put it, eventually succeeded. This however would not be a sufficient reason for chiropractic's success by itself. There were large numbers of midwives and a strong market demand, yet in their case subordination resulted.

The second effect of increases in the number of chiropractors was that it provided a crucial basis for overcoming what was obviously one of the major impediments, the lack of satisfactory training in chiropractic in Australia. Without assistance from any other source, chiropractors were faced with having to establish a training institution themselves which could then be incorporated into the tertiary education system. The 'locals' attempted to do this but with meagre resources were limited in the standard of training they could provide. The International College of Chiropractic was set up with financial assistance provided by chiropractors themselves—$1000 each per year in the first instance raised $300 000 to get the institution off the ground. Obviously only with a large number of practitioners operating (successfully) in the community could enough finance be raised to get an adequate education programme established. Furthermore, however marginal the chiropractors may have been in the earlier periods, clearly by this time they were no longer economically marginal. At no time for instance with midwives was there any suggestion that substantial amounts of money could be donated to establish a separate training institution, or indeed to finance a political campaign to avoid subordination. With a large scale expensive education programme established, chiropractors were then in a position to meet and answer most of the objections that had been raised to the registration, notably the AMA criteria set out in its science sub-committee report, and that of the Liberal party in Victoria that adequate training was not available in Victoria but only in the United States.

These then would appear to be the obvious explanations for the politico-legal legitimation of chiropractic, and are those which tend to be advanced by the chiropractors themselves. Yet in my opinion they do not fully explain its legitimation in themselves, however relevant they may be. Why, for instance, after accepting the authority of the advice of medicine for decades, was its advice discarded in the late 1970s? Medicine after all remained implacably opposed to chiropractic and still is, its accommodation of chiropractic being extremely reluctant and based as much on legal advice as to its advisability as on acceptance of the benefits of chiropractic treatment. To explain more adequately the legitimation of chiropractic then, I believe it is necessary to go beyond the explanations the chiropractors themselves give and evaluate the wider politico-ecnomic context of health care in Australian society.

From the beginning of the twentieth century the state began to play a greater role in the health system. For most of the twentieth century, however, it has delegated responsibility for health matters to its 'organic intellectuals', the medical profession, to organise the provision of health care. The phenomenon of 'medical dominance' which has been a central focus of this study has been possible, indeed a result of, state patronage for the medical profession. The authority of the expertise of medicine prevented the legitimation of chiropractic for most of the period under consideration. 'New' occupations as a result were legitimated only by the patronage of the medical profession (eg physiotherapy), and the condition of patronage (and registration) was usually subordination to medicine. Because chiropractic refused to accept even the same theory of knowledge as medicine, its attempts at legitimation were denied and exclusion operated. As state intervention increased chiropractic was able to look to the state for sponsorship rather than to the patronage of the medical profession. Commissions of inquiry were established despite medical opposition, a move which would have been unthinkable in the 1950s or even 1960s (the Western Australian experience notwithstanding).

Why then was that state prepared to recognise chiropractic even in the face of staunch medical opposition? Its own legitimacy was at stake to some extent; the fact that so many people attended chiropractors meant it could not be ignored and expected to go away. More than that however would appear to be the growing compatibility of chiropractic knowledge with dominant class interests. Medicine and chiropractic may utilise different theories of knowledge but in some major respects they can be seen to exist within the same paradigm. Medicine with its emphasis on germ theory sees ill health as an individual and biological phenomenon. Chiropractic, emphasising subluxations, sees it as individual and mechanical. Neither sees it as a social and political phenomenon and rooted in the conditions of existence of captialist society. Chiropractic if anything espouses more of an engineering approach to health than medicine does; individuals are like machines which can be tinkered with to get back into good running order. And good running order means producing surplus value.

Back injuries and strains have always been a major source of productivity loss in capitalist societies. Inglis (1978) for instance has argued that in the United Kingdom, 56 000 workers are off work on any one day with back pain at an estimated cost of 500 million dollars to the economy annually. Australian figures are not easy to come by but a study of back problems in the meat industry carried out in the 1950s found that fully half the workers examined had some ortho-paedic problem (Ward Committee Transcripts: 1679–1680). Very conservative unpublished figures calculated by the Australian Bureau of Statistics, indicate that cases of strain, sprain of the back and hernia constituted 18 per cent of all industrial accidents in the financial year 1976–1977, a loss of earnings alone (not to say value of production) of 31 million dollars, an estimated two and a half times that lost by industrial stoppages in that year.

Chiropractic treatment, it is important to note, is fused with ideological elements as well. The ideology of 'blaming-the-victim' is a common one in capitalist societies, one which focuses responsibility upon the individual without consideration of the political and economic context in which that person lives. In the occupational health and safety sphere this ideology is represented by the concept of 'accident proneness'. The responsibility for a back injury for example can be attributed to the individual who wasn't lifting properly, rather than the nature of the work process itself which may require the continual lifting of heavy objects and training in correct lifting prin-ciples. Focusing on back injuries as an individual and structural or biomechanical phenomenon, as chiropractors do, is ideological in the sense that it diverts attention away from the social and political nature of those injuries.

Furthermore, what evidence there is allows the speculation that chiropractic may in fact be better than medicine at fixing back problems incurred in industry, and thus may potentially serve dominant class interests better than doctors in this particular instance. A pilot study carried out in 1979 comparing the treatment of low back pain by chiropractors and medical practitioners in terms of work time loss and cost, found that, within certain limitations, chiropractic treatment was not only substantially cheaper but the workers returned to work more quickly than those treated by medical practitioners

(Dillon, 1979). The International Chiropractors' Association also provides evidence drawn from official sources which suggests that chiropractors are more effective in dealing with industrial back injuries (quoted in ACA, 1979). Some official recognition of this growing social control function is evidence by the registration of chiropractic services for the needs of the Workers' Compensation and Motor Accident Board.

Chiropractors of course have promoted this for a long time. The first volume of the journal of the CAV in 1959 carried an article by Mr Alan Brockhoff, Technical Director of Brockhoffs Biscuits Pty Ltd, espousing chiropractic as a form of treatment for back injuries, including his own (notably incurred when skiing however rather than at work): 'These three cases and several others I know of in the factory were despairing of getting complete relief from medical treatment. After chiropractic treatment we are all back full time.' (quoted in *Chiropractic*, May, 1959: 23)

In November 1980, an advertising sheet from a firm of chiropractors expelled from the ACA for misleading advertising, was placed in suburban letter boxes. Headed 'Attention Employees, Employers and Personnel Managers', it argued: 'It has always been our aim to assist the worker to resume work with as little as possible or no delay. This then reduces the interruption to his industrial output.' With health effectively defined as the ability to produce surplus value (that is, to work), chiropractic has been seen to be very effective. This also explains its attractiveness to the traditional middle class farming community where inability to work hard physically often results in total loss of income. Hence the support for chiropractic, from the rural Iowans which McCorkle studied and used to explain the success of chiropractic, through to the deputations from rural groups such as the Country Party and Country Women's Association for chiropractic registration. Consideration of the politico-economic context of chiropractic is thus important in explaining its politico-legal legitimation. This legitimation as we have seen was on a clinical rather than a scientific basis. The lack of scientific legitimacy in the end did not prevent the politico-legal legitimation from occurring. For some of the state subsidies which medicine had traditionally enjoyed (insurance rebates, workers' compensation treatment, repatriation and so on) to be directed at chiropractic also, it was obviously necessary to be able to distinguish between those qualified and those not.

Although chiropractic has espoused these advantages to the state for a long time, the extent of medical dominance was sufficient to prevent any serious questioning of chiropractic's exclusion. What seems to have 'tipped the balance' in favour of chiropractic was the changing dynamics of medical dominance and a growing awareness of the problems caused by back injuries, as the state became more active in post-war Australia. The need to be able to distinguish between those qualified and those not, provided the basis for the statutory recognition of chiropractic and the transformation of its position from 'exclusion' to 'limitation'.

The result of this transformation has been that chiropractors have joined the ranks of the 'organic intellectuals' of capitalist societies, becoming important agents of social control on behalf of capital in their own right. A condition of legitimation has been an abandonment of their claim to be a complete alternative system of health care. Instead they have been recognised as specialists in spinal manipulative therapy. They are 'limited' rather than 'subordinated' because they have retained their status of 'primary contact' practitioner, in other words practising without referral from a medical practitioner. The issue of chiropractic's ability to treat visceral conditions (that is, other than musculoskeletal ones) remains an open one. The 'scope of practice' issue is recognised by chiropractors themselves as an important one; while their claim to be a complete alternative system of care has been rejected, their occupational territory has not been restricted just to musculoskeletal disorders. They retain the right to treat other conditions and some clinical evidence exists to suggest their ability to successfully do so—for example in the case of migraine headaches (Parker and Tupling, 1976: 373–378). Their registration furthermore has brought them into conflict over occupational territory with other medical specialists such as radiologists, and this will be an ongoing struggle.

With legitimation achieved furthermore, some features of the medical model of development are beginning to appear, in particular further specialisation and division of labour—again, along patriarchal lines. A new health occupation is proposed—that of chiropractor's assistant, to be filled it appears mainly by women, trained not in a college of advanced education but in a technical college. The ideology of professionalism which, as I have shown, has been a major feature in the development of medicine, is being reproduced by chiropractors themsleves and subprofessional dominance is occurring.

Finally medical dominance itself, while challenged by the politico-legal legitimation of chiropractic, has emerged if not unscathed, at least intact. Chiropractic has been incorporated into the health division of labour primarily as a specialist in treatment of one part of the body. Any further claim awaits considerable research. Medicine however retains its pre-eminent position.

Conclusion

This study has examined historically the development of the social structure and organisation of health care delivery. The main feature of this development has been the progressive differentiation in the division of labour as specialisation of health work tasks has occurred. A complex division of labour has resulted, one which is differentiated not only by occupation but also by a number of other factors including gender, social class and medical knowledge held, all of which dissect the work performed in different ways. The main feature of the social organisation of health care delivery is medical dominance.

The hierarchicalisation and dominance by medicine are often explained in terms of the differential amounts of medical knowledge held by members of different occupations within the hierarchy. Such a division of labour was 'necessary' to cope with the improvements in medical knowledge of aetiological factors in disease and techniques for treating illness. Different positions in the hierarchy therefore are explained by the different amounts of control over this technology and knowledge.

I have argued against this technological determinist explanation whose adequacy is limited because it ignores the social processes involved in the development of a differentiated health labour force. In particular it is necessary to differentiate between the technology itself and the social relationships which produce that technology and evolve to cope with it. A distinction is also necessary between the technical division of labour which denotes occupational position and amount of medical knowledge held (that is, access to technology), and the social division of labour which involves social relationships resulting from an hierarchically organised social structure, tied in the last instance to the capitalist mode of production. Such an hierarchically organised social structure is organised along class and gender lines which are reproduced in microcosm within the health arena. These social relations dictate which technology is used, how and when it is used and who controls its use in health care. As I have shown historically, the hierarchy in health care developed *prior* to the development of scientific medicine. The effect of the development of scientific medicine and technology was to strengthen and extend enormously that hierarchy. Changes in knowledge and techniques occurred but only within the constraints of existing patterns of control. From this point of view, as this study has attempted to demonstrate, technology is not the driving force underlying the shape of the health care system. It is ahistorical to assume that it is so (see also Daly and Willis, 1987). The development of medical science and technology substantially affected the hierarchical health division of labour, but not to the same extent as the differentiation resulting from a pre-existing hierarchy based on class and gender factors.

Contrary to technological determinist explanations then, the argument is that class and gender relations of the wider society are reproduced within the social organisation of health care. Class interests are reflected in two ways within the health division of labour. Firstly, they are represented directly by relations of domination and subordination. Some of these are class based (power relations), others are not (authority relations). The indirect effect of class upon medical practice is reflected in the ideological component of scientific medicine. Scientific medicine as an amalgam of science and ideology promotes a view of illness and appropriate treatment that is compatible with dominant class interests. Doctors thus contribute to the promotion of bourgeois ideological hegemony in Australian capitalist society. Furthermore, it is this indirect effect of class upon medical practice which is at the root of the differentiation in the health division of labour. This indirect effect, denoted by a relationship of compatibility, is crucial to explaining the phenomenon of medical dominance. The differentiation in the division of labour must be understood in the wider politico-economic context of which the health system is a part. The essential backdrop to the study is the development of capitalism from its laissez-faire stage in the nineteenth century. Two features of this transition are relevant: the growth in intervention by the Australian capitalist State and the development of new forms of legitimacy, in particular the claim to possession of scientific knowledge. The attainment of medical dominance can only be understood with reference to these two developments.

As a number of writers have pointed out, state patronage of medicine provides one of the foundations upon which medical dominance is based. The state has intervened primarily by the provision of statutory registration legislation and medical dominance has depended upon the statutory rigidification of the occupational territories of other health occupations. Competitors have been subordinated, limited or excluded so as to maintain the dominant structural position of medicine through the patronage of the state, mainly in the form of licensing regulations which reproduce medical dominance. Indeed the division of labour in a formal sense takes shape through the struggle over licensing. As Bucher and Strauss (1961) have argued licensing legislation can be seen as the historical deposits of the exercise of power and authority.

Yet as we have seen different phases in the relationship between medicine and the state are discernible, as the state came to intervene more actively in the health arena beyond the needs of basic legitimacy. The struggle over licensing then can only be understood in terms of this wider context. This wider perspective involves the willingness of the state to accept occupational definitions of client need and institutionalise the collegiate control (see Johnson, 1972), which provided the basis for medical dominance.

Now this is not to imply a mechanistic functionalist translation of the 'requirements of capital' into legislation in the state arena. Nor is it to imply a coincidence of interests between the medical profession and the state at all times (see for instance Hunter, 1969). The relative autonomy of the state means that ideology and struggle render the sphere of legislation a problematic issue.

This is reflected in the different modes of domination over health occupations through which medical dominance is reproduced. Indeed it is of considerable interest to consider what factors govern the mode of domination which eventuates. What leads to the use of one mode rather than another? A number of factors seem to be important here.

One of these is the salience of the threat to medicine posed by work activities of other health occupations. Those occupations which compete for medicine's core work activities of diagnosis and prescription are likely to experience the most opposition. Clearly an adequate analysis of this factor would need to be based on a more complete examination of health occupations than the three presented here but a general account is possible. Chiropractic for instance claims to be a complete alternative system (to medicine) of health care, and one furthermore which negates the need for doctors at all. Hence the attempt at exclusion, the most complete form of domination. Most competing health occupations however have been subordinated. Midwifery for example has an overlapping occupational territory with both general practitioners and (later) obstetricians. Optometry on the other hand is not centrally related to diagnosis and prescription of medicine as a whole but only to one small segment. Medicine as a whole then has been half-hearted in its attempt to subordinate it and limitation has been the result. This limitation is based on 'an earlier and informal process of pre-emptive professional deskilling' so that the threatening elements in other medical roles have been actively excised (Larkin, 1978:853). In the case of optometry this would be diagnosis of ocular pathology.

Yet this 'threat' factor does not entirely explain the mode of domination which has resulted. Medicine attempted to exclude chiropractic and for many years was successful but the distribution of power in health policy determination meant that exclusion could not be sustained. As a result of the registration of chiropractic a 'lesser' (in terms of extent of medical control) mode resulted, that more closely approximated limitation. The other factor important in determining the mode of domination is labour force divisions resulting from the relations of production generally. Sexual stereotyping resulting from a patriarchal sexual division of labour is important here and may be more important in some instances than other factors such as class. The subordination of midwives by their incorporation into nursing was the result of the emergence of general practice with a claim to obstetrics as its occupational territory. The ideology of naturalism which underpins technological determinism, facilitated the subordination of midwives. Chiropractors and optometrists by contrast were overwhelmingly male and less easily subordinated. Para-medical occupations specifically created as subordinate (nurses, radiographers etc) furthermore were (and are) overwhelmingly female. The effect as Gamarnikow (1978:120) argues in relation to nurses, is that the relationship (with ideological resonances of the power relations between men, women and children in the patriarchal family) with a mode of domination resulting from the process of struggle, depends upon the specific historical conjuncture. Dentistry, for instance as Freidson (1977) shows, emerged at the same time as medicine was being unified and had staked a claim to a specific occupational territory prior to the rigid demarcation lines being drawn. The factors outlined above which are paramount in each case must be analysed historically.

Medical dominance then rests upon state patronage, achieved through medicine's role in reproducing the relations of production and seeking to maintain bourgeois ideological hegemony. Medicine however is not only a mechanism for the reproduction of the class structure but has also been a beneficiary, as control over the health field has been achieved to a considerable extent. Such control is legitimated by the ideology of professionalism; a specific form of the ideology of expertise. Professionalism is a part of the dominant ideology based on the legitimacy of science, and permits inequality by introducing differences in status throughout the medical hierarchy. Such an ideology is not static and monolithic but contradictory and changing in all situations.

Indeed, further to this, technological determinist explanations for the division of labour must also be seen as basically ideological. Technological determinism (underpinned by naturalism) is the ideological representation of the capitalist division of labour. It locates divisions in the labour process in technological imperatives resulting from the forces of production, rather than the relations of production. As such it legitimates inequality and exploitation.

The issues in wider perspective

The issues examined in this book relate to wider sociological concerns particularly with the development of the labour process. The major one of these concerns is an important one within sociology, the relationship between the differentiation in the division of labour and the emergence of a class structure. Broadly speaking two positions on this issue are evident. For Marx (1968) the existence of a polarised class structure under capitalism is integral to explaining this differentiation, whereas for Durkheim and Weber this is not the case. The progressive differentiation for Durkheim (1947) was explained by the modernisation process and is associated with the developments of science and technology. Weber (1968) on the other hand viewed differentiation in the division of labour as a feature of the process of rationalisation which all societies were undergoing regardless of the system of economic relationships by which production was organised. Rationalisation was thus expressed in changes in knowledge and differentiation in the division of labour. Both Weber and Durkheim would accept that modern society is a class society, but they differ from Marx on the pivotal role of class in explaining the division of labour.

In this study I have argued broadly speaking for the Marxian position, though in a qualified way. I have attempted to show, with reference to the health arena, that class factors were crucial to the progressive differentiation in the health division of labour. The formation of the labour process in the health arena reflects in microcosm the labour process in a capitalist social formation analysed by writers such as Braverman (1974) and Marglin (1974). Several features of the wider labour process are apparent in the social organisation of medical care. These include the concentration of theoretical knowledge in management's (that is doctor's) hands, deskilling and fragmentation of tasks and a division of labour directed towards capital accumulation control rather than efficiency (see also Daly and Willis, 1988).

Yet the Marxist position must be qualified to take greater account of gender. While class factors were crucial to the progressive differentiation in the division of labour they were not the whole story. In some historical instances, such as the subordination of midwives which is analysed here, the gender of the historical actions must also be considered.

The future of medical dominance

The analysis presented in this book is a dynamic not a static one. As we have seen, medical dominance reflects a long historical process of production and reproduction. For the purposes of this study detailed analysis of the historical process has ended in the 1930s with the attainment of 'professionalism' as the form of internal self control over the work of doctors. I have argued that this came about primarily with the granting to the Medical Board of Victoria (a body comprised entirely of doctors) full autonomy for internal regulation of the profession. With the passing of an infamous conduct clause, doctors were able to supervise the professional behaviour of their colleagues.

Sine 1945, the tendency towards state intervention in health care has increased, particularly under social democratic type Labor political governments. An attempt in the late 1940s to introduce a national health service broadly along English lines was prevented only by a High Court ruling that such a scheme would involve civil conscription of doctors, something the Australian constitution proscribes. The long period of conservative government in the 1950s and 1960s saw health care funded through private health insurance companies, a development initiated by the doctors themselves in conjunction with the government, to preserve their autonomy. This period arguably represents the heyday of medical dominance.

In the mid-1970s however the reformist Whitlam Labor government, in the teeth of medical opposition, introduced a national health insurance scheme called Medibank. It reimbursed a substantial proportion of medical fees but did not interfere with autonomy or fee-for-service payment for medical services. This scheme was wound down with a return to private health insurance under the Fraser Liberal–National Party coalition in the late 1970s and early 1980s but reintroduced in a slightly modified form by the Hawke Labor government on its election in 1983. Now called Medicare, the scheme again refunds part of the fee paid to doctors without affecting their autonomy.

Within this broad context, the historical process involving conflict with other health occupations is still ongoing. Indeed an important development in the operation of exclusion occurred while this study was in progress. This was the registration of chiropractors in 1978. As Johnson (1976b) reminds us, professionalism is an historically specific form of control over work, one with its origins in the stage of laissez-faire capitalism. The increasing role of the state in the reproduction of labour under monopoly capitalism has meant that state heteronomy has become increasingly important as an institutionalised form of occupational control.

Since the completion of this study the process has continued as medical dominance has been reproduced through contestation over occupational territories. In the case of optometry for instance there have been further negotiations over the boundaries of occupational territory between ophthalmology and optometry. In Queensland ophthalmologists have been resisting attempts by optometrists to extend their occupational territory slightly to allow them to use for diagnostic purposes of dilation, a drug currently legally restricted to use by medical practitioners. In South Australia ophthalmic interests are attempting to restrict the testing of sight by optometrists to patients over eight years of age, a move being resisted by optometrists. In the case of midwifery, negotiation continues over the appropriateness of midwives conducting home births without medical supervision, a trend being opposed by obstetrical interests. In other words the division of labour in health care continues to evolve.

The further development of the division of labour raises the issue of the likely future of medical dominance. Will medicine continue to be able to reproduce its position of dominance within the health sector? The issue has been addressed conceptually through what has come to be known as the professionalisation proletarianisation debate. A number of writers (for example Armstrong, 1976; Haug, 1973, 1975; McKinlay, nd; Oppenheimer, 1973) have analysed trends in the organisation of professional work which they see as evidence of deprofessionalisation and/or proletarianisation. These result primarily from the development of the capitalist mode of production with the increasing concentration and centralisation of capital. The trends include continuing differentiation, specialisation as a result of segmentation, and the decline in the proportion of self-employed doctors.

As analysed in this study professionalisation has been a process related to the Weberian tradition of sociological thought. It has been aimed at collective upward social mobility through social closure and monopolisation, justified by an occupational ideology (professionalism) staking a claim to autonomy and the performance of work, and in the regulation of its affairs. Deprofessionalisation then would be the opposite process, a decline in the state patronage of professionalism in particular.

The proletarianisation thesis argues that the development of capitalism, in particular the concentration and centralisation of capital, has lead to a polarisation in class terms. In the case of doctors this has been taken to mean that the petit-bourgeois class location of doctors is increasingly under threat, as evidenced in a number of ways. However the proletarianisation thesis makes most sense within an orthodox marxist position. What that position does not take adequately into account is the continued existence, even flourishing, of an intermediate class location in advanced capitalist societies, between the major historical classes of capital and labour. For this reason as outlined earlier a distinction is needed between an old or traditional middle class (small businesspersons, family farmers etc) and a new middle class comprised of major professional groups. Proletarianisation has occurred mainly to the former group. In the latter as Freidson (1977:28) has argued, self-employment or employment status per se is less important as an analytical issue than the process by which control over work is established and maintained.

Doctors, as important members of the new middle class have not been proletarianised because of their involvement in the maintenance of ideological hegemony. In the specific case of doctors the basis for state patronage lies in the role of doctors' reproduction of labour power, mediating the relationship between individuals and their bodies on one hand and the state on the other. This is after all how medicine acts as an institution of social control. From this point of view, evidence for proletarianisation of doctors would be sought in the decline in their role as organic intellectuals to the dominant class and in medicine as an institution of social control.

Contrary to both these views are the arguments put forward by Freidson (1977), who argues that it is not all clear that the proponents of the proletarianisation thesis when discussing it are talking about the same thing. The trends pointed to are real enough he argues, however they don't necessarily indicate proletarianisation. The decline in the proportion of self-employed doctors for instance he argues, is a rather mechanical indicator since the 'analytical issue is not employment or self-employment as such so much as the nature of the process by which the content, terms and conditions of work are established' (Freidson, 1977:28). Many doctors in the United States (and in Australia) are employees in a nominal sense only since they are shareholders of an incorporated practice business set up mainly for tax minimisation purposes. Furthermore he argues there is no evidence of a loss of medical dominance.

> In present day health care, a professionalised industry in which the division of labour has grown increasingly complex for fifty years or more, there is little or no evidence that physicians have been losing significant elements of their monopoly over ordering and supervising the work provided by other occupations in the division of labour. (Freidson, 1977: 28)

In the Australian context there is certainly some evidence of the sort provided by the proponents of the proletarianisation thesis. The issue is whether these constitute evidence of the decline of medical dominance. The political legitimation of chiropractic, despite active opposition from the AMA certainly constitutes a challenge to medical dominance. The significance of the AMA as the political voice of medicine has also declined with the emergence of other occupational associations such as the Doctors Reform Society, and the decision of some segments such as The Australian College of Surgeons to leave the AMA. As a result it is estimated that only around 50 per cent of all doctors in Australia belong to the AMA (*New Doctor*, No 19, 1981). Another dent in the armour of medical dominance would seem to be the decision in the early 1980s that the (Federal) Commonwealth Director General of Health, for the first time need not be medically qualified. Also there is growing non-doctor representation on state health commissions. Yet one must be cautious about concluding that medical dominance is particularly threatened. Changes in the form of medical dominance do not constitute changes in the phenomenon as a whole. Limited recognition of for instance chiropractors as specialists in spinal manipulation 'is no more the end of dominance than imperial withdrawal is the remoulding of international economic relationships' (Larkin, 1981:26). For these reasons, my contention is that medical dominance still exists though its form and operation has changed in recent years. The close identification of doctors with the state has in the past been based upon class affinities, the compatibility of medical knowledge and sympathetic governments occupying the legislative arm of the state. This provided the basis for medical dominance having peaked in the 1950s and 1960s and now plateaued but, I would argue that what evidence there is does not really indicate much of a decline and certainly not enough to justify either of the theses of deprofessionalisation or proletarianisation. In order to constitute either of these latter two processes it would be necessary to demonstrate significant diminution in one or more of the three levels at which medical dominance is sustained: autonomy, authority and medical sovereignty.

At the level of *autonomy* firstly, there appear to be a number of changes which might be considered to represent a decline in medical dominance. Doctors no longer have total control over bed allocation in many metropolitan hospitals for instance. The growth of a consumer movement, particularly the women's health movement has been important in questioning and indeed restraining the unbridled autonomy which doctors have historically enjoyed. Consumer representatives have been appointed to state bodies involving doctors (including research fund allocation committees), indeed the Victorian state government is reported to be planning legislation to appoint a consumer representative on the Medical Board of Victoria, the citadel of professional autonomy. Consumer representatives have also been incorporated with state health authorities themselves serving alongside medical officers etc.

It could be argued though that these changes, thus far at least, are fairly token. Certainly little evidence is available of any substantial impact thus far. One area of impact however, is a decline in the impact of the ideology of professionalism particularly as it involves the 'doctors know best' ideology of expertise. The political experience of organised medicines' strident opposition to the introduction of the Medibank and Medicare health insurance schemes was to reinforce the notion that the organisation of health services was essentially a political phenomenon in which doctors didn't necessarily know what was best for the rest of the populace.

Insofar as the autonomy of doctors has been affected, this is arguably more the result of intra-occupational changes rather than involving outside bodies. What appears to be occurring in the Australian health system is a concentration of power in the hands of the academically oriented specialists and away from general practitioners on one hand and even private specialists on the other. This trend has been apparent for a long time but appears to have accelerated more recently. Very few general practitioners do any surgery other than in fairly remote rural areas. As in other countries general practitioners are increasingly becoming a screening device for referral to specialists for the management of most health conditions. In the speciality fields the social relations of the increasingly sophisticated medical technologies, such as randomised control trials, concentrates power in the hands of the academic salaried specialists backed up by their technicians of one sort or another (including biostatisticians) and away from the specialists engaged in private practise who rely on the academically oriented specialists and technicians to interpret the meaning of the studies involved.

Another perceived threat to the autonomy of doctors was the national health insurance schemes Medibank and Medicare. Effective record keeping it was considered would make doctors vulnerable to charges of overservicing patients. Experience has shown however that while there have been some prosecutions for blatant overservicing, the autonomy of doctors could not reasonably have been said to be affected. Where the more effective statistical picture of servicing patterns has made an impact is pointing to regions of the country where some procedures are performed as much as seven times more often than others. In all then, at the level of autonomy, while some changes are evident, the level of personal autonomy which individual doctors experience does not seem to be greatly affected.

At the level of *authority* vis a vis other health occupations some changes are also evident. Most particularly the idea of team approach to patient care, for so long mainly ideological rhetoric, does appear to be occurring rather more, though doctors remain very much as captain of the team and there is considerable variation between rural and urban areas. In this respect I agree with Freidson's contention that 'interdependence does not necessarily corrode dominance' (1977:28). There has been a marked growth in militancy amongst paramedical groups, particularly nurses. The last few years has seen nursing largely abandon professionalism as the strategy for occupational advancement and adopt trade unionism as the preferred strategy. This has lead to a number of changes helped by a perceived nursing shortage under which circumstances state governments and hospital administrators have been prepared to improve working conditions, sometimes at the expense of doctors. In one large Melbourne hospital for instance, doctors have lost their privileged parking rights and must take their chances on finding parking places like everyone else. The consequences of such a change in approach were reflected in the state of Victoria in a seven week nursing strike at the end of 1986.

What has thrown doctor–nurse relations into sharp relief has been the process of technological innovation. One of the nurses' grievances has been that they don't get consulted about which or how the technology is introduced yet they are often required to operate it and deal with patient discomfort etc. Certainly it appears that the traditional role of nurses as 'handmaidens' to the doctors has been eroded and to that extent the doctors' authority has diminished. Many doctors spoken to will report that they are aware of needing to be much more 'careful' in their relations with nurses than previously. Changes in authority relations with other health occupations are also apparent though perhaps to a lesser extent than with nurses. Attempts by some dominated occupational groups to renegotiate their occupational territories relative to medicine have in many cases led to a swift and hostile response. Medical scientists are one such group (see Gardner and McCoppin, 1988).

Another area where it could reasonably be said that medical authority has declined is with patients vis-a-vis alternative, or what should preferably be called complementary, medicine. Utilisation of complementary practitioners such as chiropractors, osteopaths, natural therapists and practitioners of traditional Chinese medicine has been growing rapidly (Willis, 1988) even in spite of, or even perhaps because of medical opposition. Chiropractic is a good example, now with statutory registration in every part of Australia and within the state funded tertiary education system. The legitimation of chiropractic, both legally and clinically, has long been opposed by organised medicine even though it is clear that individual referral relationships have existed for a long time. Medical opposition to the statutory registration of chiropractic did not prevent it occurring largely because of the gradual process of separation of medicine and the state. Whereas traditionally legitimation was dependent upon medical approval, complementary modalities have increasingly looked directly to the state for legitimation.

Yet this decline in medical authority should not be overstated. Practitioners of complementary health care modalities have so far been largely unsuccessful in gaining access to any part of the hospital system. In fact, they have done so only in a few small private hospitals. Furthermore, a number of recommendations by government inquiries for research monies to be made available to properly investigate the efficacy of these complementary modalities have fallen on the deaf ears of medically dominated research funding bodies (see Willis, 1988). In that sense the politico-legal legitimation of chiropractic with statutory registration throughout Australia, has made very little practical difference to the social structure of health care delivery. It has given chiropractors a more secure occupational territory especially in relation to musculo-skeletal (Type M) disorders, and it has been successfully translated into substantial pecuniary rewards (see Richardson, 1984), but it has not affected the division of labour in health care.

The other health occupation sometimes considered a threat to medical dominance are health administrators who are not medically qualified. Certainly there has been a trend towards chief executives of hospitals both public and private to be non-medically qualified administrators, though this varies. Likewise there has been the trend towards corporatisation of private hospitals with the entry of several American multi-national hospital companies into Australia. The question is whether such changes of ownership and direction have led to a decline in medical dominance. My argument would be that the form of dominance has changed from overt to (relatively) subtle. Medical committees within hospitals remain very powerful. Administrators may be able to implement budget cuts of one sort and another but the medical committees have a powerful say in how this occurs. The size of the budgetary cake to be divided up might be smaller as a whole but that does not mean a redistribution in the relative size of the slices.

The same might be said of the decline in medical dominance of the state health bureaucracies. In the Victorian health commission for instance a policy of administrative regionalisation was recently implemented. All but one of the regional directors are non-medically qualified. Yet they remain heavily dependent upon medical advisory committees and limited in their ability to effect changes of a distributive nature.

This raises the issue of the third level of medical dominance; that referred to as *sovereignty* at the level of the state. As in most western capitalist economies the fiscal crisis of the state has led to attempts under pressure from dominant classes, to reduce government expenditure in 'social areas' such as health and welfare. The capitalist state has been increasingly interventionist in the era of monopoly capitalism in Australia as elsewhere. Attempts to reduce government expenditure on health care have been seen in the removal of 'cosmetic' surgery items in the schedule for which Medicare benefits are payable. Services provided by the medical profession however continue to be the only ones receiving state subsidy (optometry and some oral surgery services being the only exception). This is despite a recent review of Medicare services, to which I was an adviser, in which the major term of reference was to consider whether Medicare should cover services other than those already in the scheme. More than 50 health organisations applied to have the services provided by their members provided under Medicare. Despite some limited recommendations for extensions of the scheme; for instance pilot programmes for home births and limited involvement of chiropractors in hospitals, the recommendations have not been acted on more than two years since the committee presented its report (Medicare Benefits Review Committee, 2nd Report, 1986). Though the government probably did not want to buy into a political fight with the medical profession, in my opinion, the main reason for this inactivity is not so much because of explicit state endorsement for the preservation of medical dominance, particularly while Labor governments occupy the legislative arm of the capitalist state, but rather because of a Treasury-led insistence on restraint of government spending in the era of the fiscal crisis of the state. Any expansion of the Medicare scheme would have implications for the level of government spending. The resultant outcome has the effect of preserving the status quo and therefore preserving medical dominance of publicly funded health care services.

What it does mean however is that the state has increasingly become a terrain on which struggles over social expenditure have taken place. In the wider struggle to maintain their position, the possibility at least has emerged of coalitions between doctors and patient groups to preserve social expenditure in the face of dominant class pressure to reduce it. This appears to have been the case recently in the United Kingdom with attempts by the Thatcher Government to reduce public expenditure by dismantling the National Health Service.

For now however, at the level of the state, medical sovereignty largely continues. Medicine retains its role as an institution of social control, indeed as a number of observers have noted, this may be increasing with the increasing secularisation. Non-medical representation on state health bodies remains at this point largely tokenistic and medical certificates from doctors are required to legitimate all sorts of state benefits in the health arena. Only in the area of legitimation of absence from work for sick leave purposes has there been some erosion, with some employers accepting certificates from practitioners other than doctors.

The argument made here then is that medical dominance continues. What decline there may have been has not been sufficient to suggest that either deprofessionalisation or proletarianisation has or is occurring. Instead medical dominance has changed its form and become more subtle and indirect than previously. Changes in the form of medical dominance do not mean changes in its applicability as a whole.

Yet if there has been little evidence which satisfactorily points to the decline of medical dominance to date, its possibility cannot be discounted in the future. A number of factors would seem to be at work here. The first is the growth in state involvement in the health arena. The increasing state expenditure on health makes apparent the costs of the occupational monopoly held by medicine. To understand the likely consequences of this development it is necessary to return to the distinction made by McKinlay (1977:464–465) between the four levels of analysis necessary to understanding 'the business of medicine'. These are arranged in descending order of their determining influence as: the level of financial and industrial capital, the activity of the capitalist state, the level of medicine itself and the level of the public. Medical dominance of the division of labour in other words should not be mistaken for medical control of the health sector. At each of the higher (that is more important) levels challenges to medical dominance appear likely.

At the level of the state, the temptation in attempting to control escalating health costs, or to provide health service coverage throughout the country including geographical areas where doctors choose not to practise, is to substitute a lower paid health worker such as a 'nurse practitioner' to fulfil some of the tasks currently performed by doctors. Here the distinction made by Jamous and Peloille (1970) between technicality and indetermination is relevant. This substitution is more likely in those aspects of technicality in medical work; that is those that can be written down in manuals for others to use. Faced with this possibility, professionalism as an occupational ideology is likely to increasingly stress the more indeterminate aspects of medical work (medical mystique).

Threats to medical dominance also appear likely at the level of industrial and financial capital as mediated (in a relatively autonomous way) by the capitalist state. Medical dominance I have argued, rests upon state patronage resulting from the compatibility of medical knowledge and medical practice with dominant class interests. Professionalism as a form of work control entailing dominance in other words, was achieved by medicine when the political and economic conditions necessary to sustain it coincided with these class interests. It follows that if the political and economic conditions required to sustain medical dominance no longer exist then it is likely to be undermined. Already there is some evidence in the United States at least, of corporate opposition to the current organisation of medical care, with its enormous cost. General Motors, the world's largest corporation, is reported to spend more on health insurance for its workers than it does for steel, with the cost of health insurance adding around $100 to the cost of every vehicle produced (Brown, 1979:208). Corporate sponsored reform of medicine has already occurred in the United States with the Rockefeller and Carnegie foundation funded Flexner report (see Berliner, 1975). The historical lesson for medicine is apparent.

Furthermore, without wanting to read too much into the event, it seems noteworthy that while chiropractic achieved statutory registration in a way which basically resulted in a relationship of limitation to medicine, this limitation is not complete. The issue of 'scope of practice', that is the extent to which chiropractors are capable of treating 'organic' conditions was left open to be resolved by further struggle over occupational territories. This may reflect an interest in results suggested by chiropractors themselves that spinal manipulation may enable workers to return to work (and surplus value production) *quicker* than does conventional medical treatment. The effects of escalating health costs in the United States have led Alford (1975) to recognise (using interest group theory) an emergent struggle between what he calls 'corporate rationalisers' versus 'professional monopolists'.

Such a threat to medical dominance from financial and industrial capital on one hand and the state on the other will be facilitated paradoxically by developments in medical knowledge itself. The effects of the corporatist paradigm on medical knowledge are only just beginning to be realised. These have been detailed by Armstrong (1977). The individualist paradigm was based upon clinical experience (clinical sense) which stressed personal knowledge validated through experience. The corporatist paradigm by contrast produces medical knowledge by the 'scientific method' based upon universal knowledge. The epitome of the 'scientific method' for evaluating medical treatment is the randomised control trial. This methodological device was developed in the 1940s, initially to test the effects of various drugs (originally streptomycin in tuberculosis). Patients are randomly assigned to one of three groups, a control group which receives no treatment at all, a 'placebo' group in which the participants received treatment, medication for instance in which the active ingredient is missing, and an experimental group in which the treatment under evaluation is administered. For that treatment to be judged effective the results in the experimental group must be significantly better than those in either of the other two groups (see Cochrane, 1972).

Interpretation of the results of such trials may not require medical training and thus makes the practice of medicine potentially more accountable. It stresses the technical component and thus undermines the cherished centrepiece of professionalism. This is freedom from lay evaluation (what Friedson, 1970a, calls the 'sacred cow'). The implications of randomised control trials are thus revolutionary and not unrecognised by members of the medical profession who have on occasions refused to participate in such trials, obstructed them or to a considerable extent ignored the implications of the findings for existing practices (Cochrane, 1972:45–46). The effect of randomised control trials is thus to demystify the indeterminate aspects of medical practice and as Haug (1975) has shown, make it vulnerable to codification into a set of rules and procedures which are ripe for computerisation and easily grasped by persons without formal medical training. In this situation the ideology of professionalism is likely to become even more militant and strident, particularly from that segment of the medical profession losing out, fighting a rearguard action to stress the more indeterminate aspects of medical practice and preserve the position of the medical profession in the face of challenges to its position. This is already becoming evident in the swing to the right wing of the political spectrum which some doctors' organisations have experienced recently.

Greater accountability and technicality may be to either or both the corporate sector and the state, or the public. Codification demystifies medical practice and makes the emergence of a better informed patient populace possible as well as technically competent self-help groups who are able to draw on medical knowledge themselves. Women's health groups have been the major community group to emerge in this respect.

The future of medical dominance over the production of health care is an uncertain one then and, as the country enters the third century of white settlement, the historical process continues. If the extent of medical dominance peaked in the 1960s and has declined since then, further declines appear likely. While the hierarchy of health care workers may be dominated by medicine this does not mean medicine has overall control and challenges are occurring from three directions; from an increasingly informed and articulate public, from financial and industrial capital anxious to preserve the ability of capital accumulation and from other health workers. The last group is important. While medicine dominates the health hierarchy it is still a negotiated hierarchy in which dominated groups do struggle and not without effect.

Postscript: the politics of medical dominance

The purpose of this brief postscript is to assess the relevance of medical dominance for the provision of health care. The study having established what medical dominance is, where it came from and how it operates; the postscript considers the related question of the policy implications of such a phenomenon.

First however a caveat is necessary relating to levels of influence over the health care system. As the study has made clear dominance and control over the division of labour does not mean control over the health care system as a whole. As McKinlay (1977:464–465) makes clear with his use of the game analogy, control over the field of play is not the same as control over the whole game. Also to be taken into account are the owners of the field on which the game takes place as well as the makers of the rules of the game. In health care, or what he calls 'the business of medicine' there are four levels of analysis necessary for an adequate understanding, in descending order of their determining influence: the level of financial and industrial capital, the level of the capitalist state, the level of medicine itself and the level of the public. What sort of health care is experienced and how that care is organised then is only partially the result of specific activities of the medical profession. Illness mediates social relations in all societies. In capitalist societies it mediates the social relations of production for individuals. For the medical profession as agents of social control in that society, the requirement is to mediate for individuals, the effect of living in such a society and to consider the adverse consequences which many suffer.

But while there is much about the health field that doctors do not control, they operate in a political space cleared for and by them which has considerable consequences for the manner in which health care is provided. I would argue that the most important political consequence of medical dominance is that it prevents the most effective utilisation of health resources in society.

The health resources which are being underutilised are primarily the skills of other health workers. In order to make this argument it is necessary to consider the politics of skill. Skill is a very difficult concept to define. It must be considered a relativist concept rather than being defined as some absolute notion of precisely defined knowledge, formulas and rules. It is socially constructed at different periods. Skill as a concept varies historically; there is not much demand today for the skill of wheelwrights and coachbuilders. It also varies culturally; there is not a lot of demand or market advantage to be gained by the holders of the sorts of skills that aborigines have in this society which include living off the land. It depends very much on who is doing the defining as to what the skills are, which are considered to be appropriate. What skills are recognised and how they are recognised is a highly political process and changes over time.

In the health arena, the politics of skill are organised around the phenomenon of medical dominance with state backing and enshrined in Medicare. All statutory registration Acts for health occupations other than doctors contain a clause exempting doctors from the restrictive provisions placed on others who may practice the skills being defined in the Act. The assumption built into the health system is one of universal competence or skills on the part of the medical profession. This assumption is enshrined in Medicare, as a substantial number of the submissions made to the Layton Inquiry reviewing Medicare, in effect suggested. This is reflected in the fact that whatever goes on in the consultation between a doctor and a patient can be claimed for on Medicare. Similar treatment provided by other health care practitioners (other than optometrists) cannot. Yet it is possible in my view to make a plausible argument that in some contexts practitioners other than doctors are in fact more skilled. It is possible for instance to make a good argument that midwives are more skilled than general practitioners or obstetricians at uncomplicated deliveries; that chiropractors are better at fixing bad backs than most general practitioners; that dieticians are better at providing nutritional advice than most general practitioners; that 'lay' acupuncturists are more skilled at providing acupuncture than many members of the medical profession (general practitioners complete a very short course in acupuncture, some as short as four weeks yet 'lay' acupuncturists often study the practice for seven years). It should be noted that this argument is not made to denigrate the skills which doctors have and from which we have all benefited at various times, rather it is to argue that the skills of others are being underutilised. Medical dominance in the health arena means that we largely have medical definitions of what constitutes skill, including the skill of all other health occupations.

Medicare reimbursement is only one aspect of the phenomenon of underutilisation however. The others include medical opposition to the establishment of the better training facilities which some other

health occupations need, to their statutory registration, to their practising without medical supervision and in some cases to their very existence. As a recent document on women's health in Victoria (1987)
makes clear this restricts the choices available to consumers about
where health care is available. Many women expressed the wish to
have routine gynecological procedures (pap smears, antenatal visits)
performed by a nurse or midwife. As in most places antenatal care is
only available from midwives working under the direction of obstetricians, and places are limited, many miss out.

Medical dominance of funding bodies has meant that proposed
research into the efficacy and importantly into the limitations of some
forms of treatment has little chance of receiving support, being likely
to be considered at best as being of curiosity value.

The other major way in which medical dominance is preventing the
most effective utilisation of health resources is a more indirect one.
The effect of the hegemony of the corporatist paradigm of medical
knowledge outlined in the main study, with its individual biomedical
approach to health care, based as the study has argued on a relationship of compatibility with (dominant) class interests, has directed emphasis away from the *social* causation of disease, from prevention,
public, environmental and occupational health. Instead through promotion of the direction of research, and funding of such research,
medical dominance has been responsible to a considerable extent for
an orientation to health which lacks an holistic commitment to providing health care in the context of the lives people lead, relying often
instead upon a 'victim blaming' individualisation of health problems.
While of course there are many members of the medical profession in
the forefront of the social health movement, the overall effect of
medical dominance has been to encourage a view that health problems
can be solved best by more of the same and that more resources spent
on research within this paradigm will eventually yield technological
and individualist solutions.

Furthermore as most doctors originate from a fairly limited spectrum of the population (anglo-celtic, male, middle class), medical
dominance also means that the awareness of influences on health from
social causes such as class, ethnicity, gender, where people live and
what sort of work they do, is thereby limited.

In the face of perceived threats to medical dominance, the ideological rearguard action to preserve it has often had the effect of
restricting socially progressive legislation. Such an instance was the recent attempt by the Victorian government to respond to consumer
demands for greater accountability of doctors, to establish an independent health services complaints office with investigative and
conciliation functions separate to the doctor dominated registration
board; in other words a source of accountability outside the medical

profession. Medical opposition to the bill resulted in a substantial dilution of its provisions, including the loss of investigative functions where the registration board had jurisdiction (see Willcox and Ednie, 1987).

Despite the ease of demonstrating that many medical decisions are made as much on social and moral grounds as they are on technical grounds, the 'ideology of expertise', the view that 'the doctor and only the doctor knows best' continues. Against that view which encourages a sort of apolitical passivity on the part of consumers, a definite trend is discernible. Consumer groups have grown up in many areas of the health system; some specifically organised around particular medical conditions, others espousing more general advocacy. The emergence of the social/environmental/public/occupational health movements, including as they do many socially progressive members of the medical profession is another indication. The challenges to medical dominance and the rearguard action being fought to preserve it are indicative of a social process towards *empowerment* of individuals in relation to their health.

Methodological appendix

This brief appendix examines some of the methodological issues associated with the study. The task of analysing the dynamics of medical dominance has been facilitated by a considerable tradition of medico-historical research in the state of Victoria. Yet a critical stance has been adopted towards much of this tradition. To utilise a distinction made by Hicks (1982) it is basically *medical history* rather than the *history of medicine*. Several objections can be raised to this tradition of medical history. As Freidson (1970a: 13) has argued much of medical history is about medical discoveries and discoverers from the present day perspective of 'valid' medical knowledge. By not examining 'everyday medical work they fail to communicate how radically different from today the everyday work of the practitioner was'.

Such accounts have a positivistic methodological basis, which can also be challenged: 'There is great concern with the solid facts of scientific and medical discovery and a belief that a careful, well documented scholarly approach will reveal even truer information and an even more complete record.' (Figlio, 1977: 264)

Figlio goes on to argue that serious objection can be raised to this approach on epistemological grounds as being empiricist:

the concrete record of scientific and medical development assumes without question that there are solid facts to discover and that the continual discovery of these facts leads eventually to the state of knowledge that we have today. But this very assumption automatically isolates the endeavour called 'scientific' or 'medical' advancement from its social context. That is, it neither examines the non-intellectual contingencies which mould ideas, nor does it look at the use of scientific or medical concepts as cultural, social, religious or ideological tools. By their very definition facts could never carry this kind of load. It is my belief therefore, that the solid record of the history of medicine, with its cautious abstinence from interpretation or evaluation, is deceptive, because it reinforces in an implicit and unimpeachable way the currently held views of medicine and does this in the name of 'historical perspective'. (Figlio, 1977: 265)

The effects of such an approach to medical history when carried to an extreme become evident, as this statement by well-known Australian scientist, Sir MacFarlane Burnett (1952: 802) indicates: 'It is hardly too much to say that no major discovery destined to be fully incorporated into established knowledge and techniques is made more than a year or two before it is inevitable.'

The tradition of the *social* history of medicine began with Sigerist (1951) and Rosen (eg 1973). This approach focuses not narrowly on medical discoveries and the 'great men' of medical science as others had tended to do but on medicine in its wider social context. It looked at how medicine was socially organised, why discoveries took place and the history of the medical profession itself. From this tradition developed a more strictly sociological approach to the study of medical history, known as the 'Leicester School'. These writers (Holloway, 1966; Jewson, 1976; and Waddington, 1977) analysed the historical sociology of medicine, though the field has remained a relatively undeveloped one until very recently with the appearance of the work of Armstrong (eg 1976), Donnison (1977), and that of Woodward and Richards (1977). Actually not only have historical accounts of medicine been medico-centric but so also have sociological accounts. The sociology of health developed from practical rather than theoretical concerns and developed its' sense of problem, many of its assumptions and some of its methods from medicine (see Willis, 1982).

This present study falls with this developing tradition of the social history of medicine. It is an historically informed sociological account in which the theoretical ideas provide the foundations and scaffolding around which the specific historical instances can be ordered. The historical analysis investigates dynamics of social change, complete with contradictions, rather than simply investigating the past in search of 'origins'. As Wright (1978; 13) argues:

> While it is true that an historical investigation will typically involve gathering data from the past, the crucial issue is not the temporality of the data, but the way in which they are analysed. It is entirely possible to conduct ahistorical investigations of the past and historical investigations of the present.

In other words while assuming the primacy of the object of study, 'facts' do not speak for themselves. Historical accounts are produced from negotiations between theoretical assumptions, concepts and methods which derive from a theoretical position, *and* from available evidence which has a demonstrable existence independent of the theory. The study in other words is not just an illustration or refinement of the theory but an attempt to explain and understand what actually occurred. Outlining concepts and defining terms then is not specifying what is to be found in the historical materials nor does it provide a basis for rejecting disconfirmatory evidence, but instead outlines the theoretical foundations on which the historiographic analysis can be constructed.

The scope of the study needed to analyse and attempt to account historically for the phenomenon of medical dominance was necessarily very broad. For this reason while some of the research is original in nature, the bulk of it has involved secondary analysis of existing sources. In using secondary analyses, as much of the original sources of evidence as could be checked was done so. In some cases, given the original narrowness, the arguments made were cast and recast, often to suit a different purpose.

The 'data' was collected from two sources. One involved content analysis of documents, legislation, journals and other historical evidence of a written nature. The other involved interviewing or oral histories of what Gorden (1975) calls 'special respondents'. These are respondents selected because their social or occupational position enables them to give information directly relevant to the study's objecives. In this study, these were participants in the actual process of reproduction of medical dominance. Some 30 interviews were recorded, all with participants in the more recent struggles involving medicine with optometry and chiropractic. In some cases it was necessary to preserve the anonymity of the respondents. An attempt was made also to interview participants from both 'sides' of the struggles.

Two problems exist with the interpretation of the evidence gained. The first is the technical nature of the issues involved which makes it difficult for the social scientist to judge the relative merits of the different therapies involved. No attempt has been made to do that. Differences over theraphy however become differences between therapists and thus the researcher is able to concentrate upon two sorts of relationships: one between practitioners, and the other between the professional associations into which the various practitioners are organised. The 'data' then is the non-technical evidence concerning the evolution of the medical profession and its relationship with other health occupations.

The second problem is what Deising (1971) calls the 'contextual validity' of the evidence gained. Given the intense political struggles which have been analysed and the rhetoric which has flowed, the difficulty is in assessing the validity of information gained, especially when actual evidence to substantiate allegations made by both sides (for example of political influence over the legislative process) is difficult to obtain. Assessing the contextual validity of evidence involves assessing each piece of evidence in the context of other pieces of evidence. This can be done in three different ways; comparing reports of events given in one interview with that given in another interview, comparing interview information with documentary evidence of the same event, and comparing document with document.

The theoretical scaffolding used to order and analyse the historical evidence rests upon structuralist foundations and this is reflected in two main ways. The first of these is the epistemological distinction between 'appearances' and 'reality', one made

> not to discuss appearances but rather to provide a basis for their explanation. The central claim is that the vast array of empirical phenomena immediately observable in social life can only be explained if we analyse the social reality hidden behind those appearances. (Wright, 1978: 12)

The historical investigation then is concerned with the level of appearances; legislation, meetings, lobbying etc, well documented in the tradition of medico-historical research mentioned previously. These appearances however derive from and are the effects of underlying structures, contradictory, fragmented and subject to transformation by struggle (such as class and gender) but essential nonetheless to the explanation of the appearances. The result is a structural explanation not a 'causal' one. A major underlying reality to the study here is capitalism. To argue structurally is to argue that capitalism is a condition of existence for the development of the division of labour in health care. It is not to argue, 'causally', that capitalism caused the development. For this reason the extent to which the analysis here can be generalised to other capitalist countries is limited. Capitalism provides no more than a condition of existence, the actual historical conjunctures involving health have been worked out differently. For this reason (as well as limitations of length) I have avoided addressing comparative issues in other countries since the medicine/capitalism nexus may have been resolved differently elsewhere. The historical evidence relates mainly to the state of Victoria and while the broad processes analysed would seem to have applied elsewhere in Australia, points of detail make wholesale generalisation hazardous.

The other effect of arguing structurally is to defend the analysis against a charge of 'doctor-bashing'. There has been a tendency within the sociology of health, using individualist assumptions to focus on individual actors or agents, so that the nature of the system is seen as one of conflict resolution between actors and groups of actors where the nature of conflict results from personalities and motivation of the actors involved. This easily leads to a type of conspiracy theory and has resulted in the charge levelled at sociologists of health that they are 'doctor bashing', which was as one medical writer put it 'until recently a harmless sport in which all could join, especially other doctors, has become institutionalised and is now called medical sociology' (Backett, quoted in Fenwick, 1978: 2).

My concern here rather is to move beyond the level of the actors involved such as doctors, to argue structurally, that is to relate the activities of doctors to the broader structural processes which impinge them. Like most individuals, doctors arc neither saints nor devils, but act within the political, social and economic space cleared for and by them in a capitalist society. The behaviour and dynamics of actors in the health system must be understood in terms of the overall political and economic framework in our society, including their class and gender positions. Likewise when discussing political activities of occupational associations such as the Australian Medical Association (AMA) the study does not focus at the level of the individuals concerned; of course the position they occupy forces them into more extreme position. What I am interested in its how the AMA operates as a medical institution.

Bibliography

Manuscripts and other unpublished sources

Bane, L. *Nurses Notebook* La Trobe Library MSS 9871.
Allen, H.B. *Private Papers* Melbourne University Archives.
Australian College of Optometry *Council Minutes* 1940–1945 Department of Optometry Library, Melbourne University.
Chief Secretary's Office Registry Book of Letters Inwards
—— Individual Files
—— Index of Letters Received
—— (Various 1870–1912—held in Public Records Office, Melbourne).
Eye, Ear and Throat Section BMA (Vic.) *Minutes* 1912–1922, held in RACO Archives, Eye and Ear Hospital, Melbourne.
Melbourne University Archives *List of Principal Benefactions* Pamphlet, 1959.
—— *Medical Faculty Minutes*, 1862–1940.
—— *Melbourne University Calendars*.
Snell, E. *Diary 1849–1859* La Trobe Library MSS 8970.
Springthorpe, J. *Diaries, 1883–1933* La Trobe University MSS 9898.
Wakefield, G. *Letters to His Family 1853–69 and 1887–88* La Trobe Library MSS 6331.
Willis, M. and R. *A Joint Autobiography* La Trobe Library MSS 9877.

Official Published Sources

Australian Bureau of Statistics (1975) *Chronic Illnesses, Injuries and Impairments*, May 1974 Ref. Paper No. 17–16, Canberra Commonwealth of Australia *Census* 1901, 1911, 1921, 1933.
—— (1980) *Handbook of Health Manpower*.
—— *Parliamentary Papers* 'Committee Concerning Causes of Death and Invalidity in the Commonwealth: Report on Maternal Mortality in Childbirth' V, 1917–1919: 997–1014.
—— *Parliamentary Papers* 'Report of the Royal Commission on Health' 4, 2, 1926–1928: 1247–1370.
Medicare Benefits Review Committee, (1986) *2nd Report*, (the Layton Report), June, Canberra: Australian Government Publishing Service.
Report of the Commission of Inquiry (1979) *Chiropractic in New Zealand*.
New South Wales *Parliamentary Papers* 'Royal Commission on the Decline of

the Birth Rate and on the Mortality of Infants in New South Wales' IV, 1904: 791.

Report of the Honorary Royal Commission Appointed to Enquire into the Provisions of the Natural Therapies Bill 1961 (The Guthrie Report).

Report of the Committee on the Future of Tertiary Education in Australia to the Australian Universities Commission II, August 1964 (The Martin Report).

Report from the Victorian Legislature Joint Select Committee on Osteopathy, Chiropractic and Naturopathy 1975 (The Ward Report).

Report of the Committee of Inquiry into Chiropractic, Osteopathy, Homeopathy and Naturopathy (The Webb Report) Canberra: Australian Government Publishing Service, 1977.

Victoria *Acts of Parliament.*

—— *Census* 1861, 1871, 1881, 1891.

—— *Parliamentary Debates.*

Victoria *Parliamentary Papers*: 'Final Report of the Royal Commission to Inquire into and Report upon the Sanitary Conditions of Melbourne' 2, 1890.

—— 'First General Report by Professor H.B. Allen, M.D.' 3, 1891.

—— 'Report of the Minister for Public Instruction, Appendix: Report on Medical Inspection and Kindred Subjects' 1910-1922.

Unpublished theses

Berliner, H. (1977) Philanthropic Foundations and Scientific Medicine, Doctor of Science, John Hopkins University.

Fett, I. (1975) Australian Medical Graduates, 1920-1972, PhD, Monash University.

Hunter, T. (1969) The Politics of National Health, Ph.D. Australian National University.

Lewis, M.J. (1976) Population or Perish: Aspects of Infant and Maternal Health in Sydney, 1870-1939, PhD, Australian National University.

McGrath, A.G. (1975) The Evolution of Medical Associations in Terms of the Concurrent Social Conditions, PhD, Sydney University.

Pensabene, T. (1979) The Rise of the General Practitioner in Victoria, 1870-1930, MEc, Monash University.

Scotton, R.B. (1970) Medical Care and Health Insurance in Australia, PhD, Melbourne University.

Thame, C. (1974) Health and the State, PhD, Australian National University.

Willis, E. (1976) The Consequences of Bureaucratization: A Study of the Work Settings of the General Medical Practice Profession, MA, Victoria University of Wellington.

Books and articles

Acknerknecht, E. (1948) 'Anticontagionism Between 1821 and 1867' *Bulletin of History of Medicine* 22, 5: 562-93.

Alford, R. (1975) *Health Care Politics: Ideological and Interest Group Barriers to Reform* Chicago: University of Chicago Press.

Allan, R.M. (1928) 'Report on Maternal Mortality and Morbidity in the State of Victoria' *Medical Journal of Australia*, 2 June: 668–85.

American Medical Association (1961) 'Medical Care for Eye Patients: Report of the Subcommittee to Study the Relations of Medicine to Optometry' *Journal of the Australian Medical Association* 178, 5.

Anderson, C.E. (1951) *The Story of Bush Nursing in Victoria* Melbourne: Renown Press.

Andrew, R. (1979) 'Graduation is the End of the Beginning' *Chiropractic College News* 5, 2: 2–3.

Armstrong, D. (1975) The Changing Basis of Medical Knowledge, unpublished paper, Unit of Sociology, Guy's Hospital Medical School.

—— (1976) 'The Decline of Medical Hegemony: A Review of Government Reports during the N.H.S.' *Social Science and Medicine* 10: 157–63.

—— (1977) 'Clinical Sense and Clinical Science' *Social Science and Medicine* 11: 588–601.

—— (1979) 'The Emancipation of Biographical Medicine' *Social Science and Medicine* 13: 1–8.

Armstrong, M. (1951) 'A Brief History of the First 50 Years of the Royal Victorian College of Nursing, 1901–1951' *Una Nursing Journal* Jubilee Issue 49: 186–215.

Armstrong, W. (1939) 'The Infant Welfare Movement in Australia' *Medical Journal of Australia* 28 October: 641–8.

Atkinson, P., Reid, M. and Sheldrake, P. (1977) 'Medical Mystique' *Sociology of Work and Occupations* 4, 3: 243–80.

Attiwill, K.G. (1965) Opthalmology and Optometry: Aspects of Vision Care. A Submission to the Federal Council of the Australian Medical Association, Carlton, Victoria: Australian Optometrical Association (mimeographed).

Australian Chiropractors Association (Victorian Branch) (1971) Analysis of AMA Paper Entitled Registration of Chiropractors Dated August 29, 1967, as Presented by the ACA (Victorian Branch) to the Honourable John F. Rossiter MP, Minister of Health, 21 June, ACA Archives.

—— (1974a) Brief to the Select Committee of Inquiry into Osteopathy, Chiropractic and Naturopathy, ACA Archives, October.

—— (1974b) *Chiropractors Draft Registration Bill*, ACA Archives.

—— (undated but published 1976) *Rebuttal to the Victorian Report upon Osteopathy, Chiropractic and Naturopathy* Bundoora, Victoria: PIT Press, ACA Archives.

Australian Chiropractors Association (1978) A Submission on Chiropractic Course Siting to the Ad Hoc Committee on Chiropractic of the VIC, ACA Archives.

—— (1979) Supplementary Brief by the Australian Chiropractors' Association to the South Australian Government Committee to Report on the Rehabilitation and Compensation of Persons Injured at Work, ACA Archives.

Australian College of Optometry (1974) *Optometry in the Australian Health Services* (edited by J. Fair) Sydney: Beaver Press.

Australian Medical Association (Victorian Branch) (1966) 'Report on Chiropractic' Supplement to *Australian Medical Association (Victoria) Monthly Paper* 48, August.

—— (1973) 'Chiropractic 1973' Supplement to *Australian Medical Association (Victoria) Monthly Paper* 118, March.

—— (1974) Brief to Select Committee of Inquiry into Osteopathy, Chiropractic, Naturopathy, ACA Archives.

—— (1976) 'Comments of the Australian Medical Association (Victorian Branch) on some Aspects of the Report from the Osteopathy, Chiropractic and Naturopathy Committee' *Australian Medical Association (Victoria) Monthly Paper* July.

Australian Physiotherapy Association (1973) *A Physiotherapy Case Against Chiropractic* ACA Archives.

Bailey, E. and Singer, C. (1964) The Public Welfare and the Profession of Optometry, unpublished paper, American Optometry Association.

Balint, M. (1964) *The Doctor, His Patient and the Illness* 2nd edn, London: Pitman Medical.

Barrett, E. (1923) 'Is the Motherhood of Australia Getting Best Value from the Maternity Bonus' *Health* 1, 5: 721–6.

Barrett, M. (1980) *Women's Oppression Today: Problems in Marxist Feminist Analysis* London: New Left Books.

Begun, J.W. (1979) 'The Consequences of Professionalisation for Health Services Delivery: Evidence from Optometry' *Journal of Health and Social Behaviour* 20, 4: 376–86.

Bell, D. (1970) *End of Ideology* New York: Free Press.

Bellaby, P. and Oribabor, P. (1977) 'The Growth of Trade Union Consciousness Among General Hospital Nurses Viewed as a Response to Proletarianisation' *Sociological Review* 25, 4: 801–22.

Berlant, J. (1975) *Profession and Monopoly: A Study of Medicine in the United States and Great Britain* Berkeley: University of California Press.

Berliner, H. (1975) 'A Larger Perspective on the Flexner Report' *International Journal of Health Services* 5, 4: 573–92.

Blackburn, R. (1969) 'A Brief Guide to Bourgeois Ideology' in Cockburn, A. and Blackburn, R. (eds) *Student Power* Harmondsworth: Penguin: 163–213.

Blainey, G. (1958) *A Centenary History of the University of Melbourne* Melbourne: Melbourne University Press.

—— (1966) *The Tyranny of Distance: How Distance Shaped Australia's History* Melbourne: Sun Books.

Bloor, M. and Horobin, G. (1975) 'Conflict and Conflict Resolution in Doctor-Patient Interaction' in Cox, C. and Mead, S. (eds) *Sociology of Medical Practice* London: Collier Macmillan: 271–84.

Boven, R., et al. (1977a) 'New Patients to Alternative Health Care' in *Report of Committee of Inquiry into Chiropractic, Osteopathy, Homeopathy and Naturopathy* Canberra: Australian Government Publishing Service: 298–364 (Western Report No. 1).

—— (1977b) 'A Study of Alternative Health Care Practitioners' in *Report of Committee of Inquiry into Chiropractic, Osteopathy, Homeopathy and Naturopathy* Canberra: Australian Government Publishing Service: 364–421 (Western Report No. 2).

—— (1977c) 'Current Patients of Alternative Health Care: A Three City Study' in *Report of the Committee of Inquiry into Chiropractic, Osteopathy, Homeopathy and Naturopathy* Canberra: Australian Government Publishing Service: 422–522 (Western Report No. 3).

Bowden, K.M. (1974) *Doctors and Diggers on the Mount Alexander Gold-*

fields Maryborough: Hedges and Bell.

Braverman, H. (1974) *Labour and Monopoly Capital: The Degradation of Work in the Twentieth Century* New York: Monthly Review Press.

Bray, S.D. (1939) 'The First Use of Radium Needles in Australia' *Medical Journal of Australia*, 3 June: 849.

Breen, A.C. (1977) 'Chiropractors and the Treatment of Back Pain' *Rheumatology and Rehabilitation* 16: 46–53.

British Medical Association (Victoria) Eye and Eye Section (1913) 'The Case Against the Proposed "Bill for the Registration of Sight-testing Opticians"' *Australian Medical Journal*, 23 August: 1102–83.

British Medical Association (Victoria) (1935) *The Book of Melbourne, Australia* Sydney: Australasian Medical Publishing Company.

Broom, L., Duncan-Jones, P., Jones, F. and McDonnell, P. (1979) *Investigating Social Mobility* Canberra: Australian National University Monograph.

Brown, A.E. (1926) 'The Position of Public Hospitals in Relation to the Medical Profession' *Medical Journal of Australia*, 9 October: 476–80.

Brown, C. (1973) 'The Division of Labours: Allied Health Professions' *International Journal of Health Services* 3, 3: 435–44.

Brown, E.R. (1976) 'Public Health in Imperialism: Early Rockefeller Programs at Home and Abroad' *American Journal of Public Health* 66: 897–903.

—— (1979) *Rockefeller Medicine Men: Medicine and Capitalism in America* Berkeley: University of California Press.

Brown, K.M. (1937) *Medical Practice in Old Parramatta* Sydney: Angus Robertson.

Browne, D.D. (1976) *The Wind and the Book: Memoirs of a Country Doctor* Melbourne: Melbourne University Press.

Bruck, L. (1893) 'The Present State of the Medical Profession in Australia, Tasmania and New Zealand' *Australasian Medical Gazette* March: 94–7.

—— (ed.) (1896) *The Sweating of the Medical Profession by the Friendly Societies in Australia* Sydney: L. Bruck Medical Publishers.

Bucher, R. and Strauss, A. (1961) 'Professions in Process' *American Journal of Sociology* 66: 325–34.

Burnet, Sir M. (1952) 'The Seeds of Time: The Impact of Microbiology on Human Affairs Since Lister's Day' *Medical Journal of Australia* 14 June: 801–6.

Butlin, N.G. (1962) *Australian Domestic Product, Investment and Borrowing, 1861–1938/39* Cambridge: Cambridge University Press.

Cambridge, A. (1903) *Thirty Years in Australia* London: Methuen.

Campbell, J. (1929–30) 'Maternal and Child Welfare in Australia' *Commonwealth Parliamentary Papers* II: 1523–4.

Campbell, S. (1980) Chiropractic and the Politics of Professionalisation, unpublished paper presented to SAANZ Conference, Hobart.

Carchedi, G. (1977) *On the Economic Identification of Social Classes* London: Routledge and Kegan Paul.

Carr-Saunders, A.M. and Wilson, P.A. (1933) *Professions* London: Oxford University Press.

Carter, R. (1958) *The Doctor Business* New York: Doubleday.

Castiglioni, A. (1958) *A History of Medicine* New York: Alfred Knope.

Chalmers, A.F. (1976) *What is This Thing Called Science?* St. Lucia: Queensland University Press.

Chambliss, W. (ed.) (1969) *Crime and the Legal Order* New York: McGraw-Hill.

Champness, R. (1952) *A Short History of the Worshipful Company of Spectacle Makers up the Beginning of the Twentieth Century*,Pamphlet, London: Worshipful Company of Spectable Makers.

Chubin, D. and Studer, K. (1978) 'The Politics of Cancer' *Theory and Society* 6, 1: 55-74.

Clarke, J., Connell, I. and McDonough, R. (1977) *On Ideology*London: Hutchison.

Cochrane, A. (1972) *Effectiveness and Efficiency: Random Reflections on Health Services* London: Nuffield Provincial Hospitals Trust.

Cole, G.E. (1950) 'The History of Infant Welfare Services in Victoria' *Una Nursing Journal* 48, July.

Collingwood History Committee (1979) *In Those Days—Collingwood Remembered* Melbourne: Richmond Hill Press.

Connell, R. (1977) *Ruling Class, Ruling Culture* Melbourne: Cambridge University Press.

—— (1979a) 'The Concept of Role and What do Do With It' *Australian and New Zealand Journal of Sociology* 15, 3: 7-17.

—— (1979b) 'A Critique of the Althusserian Approach to Social Class' *Theory and Society* 8, 3: 303-46.

Connell, R. and Irving, T. (1979) *Class Structure in Australian History* Sydney: Longman.

Craig, C. (1950) 'The Egregious Dr. Beaney of the Beaney Scholarships' *Medical Journal of Australia* 1: 593-8.

Crellin, J.K. (1968) 'The Dawn of the Germ Theory: Particles, Infection and Biology' in Poynter, F. (ed.) *Medicine and Science in the 1860's* London: Wellcome Institute of History of Medicine: 57-76.

Cresswell, D. (1897) 'Report on Diptheria in Hawthorn' *Victorian Parliamentary Papers* 2: 1775-98.

Croll, D.G. (1924) 'The Cinderella of Medicine' *Medical Journal of Australia* 27 December: 673:7.

Cummins, C.J. (1969) 'The Administration of Medical Services in New South Wales, 1788-1885' *Australian Studies of Health Service Administration* 9: 1-93.

Cumpston, J.H.L. (1927) *The History of Diptheria, Scarlet Fever, Measles, Whooping Cough in Australia, 1788-1925* Canberra: Commonwealth Department of Health.

—— (1978) *The Health of the People* Canberra: Roebuck.

Cyriax, J. (1973) 'Registration of Chiropractors' *Medical Journal of Australia* 1: 1165.

Dahrendorf, R. (1959) *Class and Class Conflict in Industrial Society* London: Routledge and Kegan Paul.

Daly, J., and Willis, E. (1987) 'The social relations of medical technology: implications for technology assessment and health policy.' in Daly, J., Green, K., and Willis, E. *Technologies in Health Care: Policies and Politics,* Canberra: Australian Government Publishing Service 2-18.

—— (1988) 'Technological innovation in health care' in Willis, E. (ed.)

Technology and the Labour Process: Australasian Case Studies Sydney: Allen and Unwin, 113–127.

Davidson, A. (1968) *Antonio Gramsci: The Man, His Ideas* Sydney: Australian Left Review Publications.

—— (1977) *Antonio Gramsci: Towards an Intellectual Biography* London: Merlin Press.

Davidson, G. (1968) *Medicine Through the Ages* London: Methuen.

Davies, C. (1979a) 'Organisation Theory and the Organisation of Health Care: A Comment on the Literature' *Social Science and Medicine* 13A: 413–22.

—— (1979b) 'Comparative Occupational Roles in Health Care' *Social Science and Medicine* 13A: 515–21.

Davison, G. (1978) *The Rise of Marvellous Melbourne* Melbourne: Melbourne University Press.

Deising, P. (1971) *Patterns of Discovery in the Social Sciences* Chicago: Aldine.

Dewdney, J.C. (1972) *Australian Health Services* Sydney: John Wiley.

Dickens, C. (1871) *The Life and Adventures of Martin Chuzzlewit* London: Chapman and Hall.

Dickey, B. (1974) 'Colonial Bourgeoisie—Marx in Australia? Aspects of a Social History of N.S.W., 1856–1900' *Australian Economic History Review* 14, March: 20–36.

—— (1977) 'Health and the State in Australia, 1788–1977' *Journal of Australian Studies* 2, November: 50–63.

Dillon, R. (1979) 'A Comparative Study of the Treatment of Lower Back Pain by Chiropractors and Medical Physicians in Terms of Work Time and Treatment Cost' Appendix A to *Supplementary Brief by the Australian Chiropractors' Association to the South Australian Government Committee to Report on the Rehabilitation and Compensation of Persons injured at Work* (originally an under-graduate paper, University of New England, Armidale, 1979).

Donnison, J. (1977) *Midwives and Medical Men* London: Heinemann.

Doran, M. and Newell, D. (1975) 'Manipulation in Treatment of Low Back Pain' *British Medical Journal* 2 April: 161–2.

Doyle, A.C. (1903) *The Stark Munro Letters* New York: Munro.

Duke-Elder, S. (1957) 'The History of Ophthalmology in Britain' *Suppl. Ad. Ophthalmalogica* 134: 24–9.

Durkheim, E. (1947) *The Division of Labour in Society* Glencoe: Free Press.

—— (1957) *Professional Ethics and Civic Morals* London: Routledge Kegan Paul.

Eddy, C.E. (1946) 'The Fiftieth Anniversary of the Discovery of X rays' *Medical Journal of Australia* 2 February: 138–44.

Ehrenreich, B. and English, D. (1973) *Witches, Midwives and Nurses: A History of Women Healers* Old Westbury, New York: Feminist Press.

Etzioni, A. (ed.) (1969) *The Semi Professions and Their Organisation* New York: Free Press.

Featonby, H.N. (1935) 'Health Administration in Victoria, 1834–1934' *Health Bulletin (Victoria)* 42: 1180–94.

Fenwick, P. (1978) Sociologists and Health System: Justice for Whom? unpublished paper presented to SAANZ Conference, Brisbane, May.

Fielding, A. and Portwood, D. (1980) 'Professions and the State—Towards a Typology of Bureaucratic Professions' *Sociological Review* 28, 1: 23–53.

Figlio, K. (1977) 'The Historiography of Scientific Medicine: An Invitation to the Human Sciences' *Comparative Studies in Sociology and History* 19, 3: 262–86.

Fishbein, M. (1925) *The Medical Follies* New York: Boris and Liverlight. light.

Fisk, J. (1980) 'A Controlled Trial of Manipulation in a Selected Group of Patients with Low Back Pain Favouring One Side' *Journal of Manipulative and Physiological Therapeutics* 3, 2: 20–4.

Foroes, T. (1966) *The Midwife and the Witch* New Haven: Yale University Press.

—— (1971) 'The Regulation of English Midwives in the Eighteenth and Nineteenth Centuries' *Medical History* 15, October: 352–62.

Ford, E. (1976) *Bibliography of Australian Medicine, 1790–1900* Sydney: Sydney University Press.

Forster, F.M. (1965) 'Mrs. Howlett and Dr. Jenkins: Listerism and Early Midwifery Practice in Australia' *Medical Journal of Australia* 25 December: 1047–54.

—— (1967) *Progress in Obstetrics and Gynaecology in Australia* Sydney: Sands.

Fosdick, R. (1952) *The Story of the Rockefeller Foundation* New York: Harper and Brothers.

Foucault, M. (1973) *The Birth of the Clinic* London: Tavistock.

Fowler, R. (1951) 'The R.H. Fetherston Memorial Lecture: Populating the Antipodes, or Migration, Motherhood and Midwifery in the Making of Victoria' *Medical Journal of Australia* 21 July: 69–75.

Frankenberg, R. (1974) 'Functionalism and After? Theory and Developments in Social Science Applied to the Health Field' *International Journal of Health Services* 4, 3: 411–27.

Freidson, E. (1970a) *Professional Dominance: The Social Structure of Medical Care* Chicago: Aldine.

—— (1970b) *Profession of Medicine* New York: Dodd Mead.

—— (1973) 'Professionalisation and Organisation of Middle Class Labour in Post Industrial Society' in Halmos, P. (ed.) Professionalisation and Social Change Social Review Monograph No. 20: 47–60.

—— (1976) 'The Division of Labour as Social Interaction' *Social Problems* 23 February: 304–13.

—— (1977) 'The Futures of Professionalisation' in Stacey, M. et al. (eds) *Health and the Division of Labour* London: Croom Helm: 14–40.

Gamarnikow, E. (1978) 'Sexual Division of Labour: The Case of Nursing' in Kuhn, A. and Wolpe, A. (ed.) *Feminism and Materialism* London: Routledge & Kegan Paul: 96–123.

Gandevia, B.H. (1948) *The Melbourne Medical Students, 1862–1942* Melbourne: Melbourne Medical Students Society.

—— (1952) 'A Review of Victoria's Early Medical Journals' *Medical Journal of Australia* 9 August: 184–91.

—— (1953) 'William Thomson and the History of the Contagionist Doctrine in Melbourne' *Medical Journal of Australia* 21 March: 398–403.

—— (1954) 'John Thomas Rudall F.R.C.S. (1828–1907): His Life and Journal

for the Year 1858' *Medical Journal of Australia* 25 December: 989–1046.
—— (1957) *An Annotated Bibliography of the History of Medicine in Australia* Sydney: Australasian Medical Publishing Company.
—— (1960) 'Land, Labour and Gold: The Medical Problems of Australia in the Nineteenth Century' *Medical Journal of Australia* 14 May: 753–62.
—— (1967) 'Medical History in its Australian Environment' *Medical Journal of Australia* 2: 941–6.
—— (1971) 'The Medico-Historical Significance of Young and Developing Countries, Illustrated by Australian Experience' in Clarke, E. (ed.) *Modern Methods in the History of Medicine* London: Althone Press.
—— (1978) *Tears Often Shed* Sydney: Pergamon.
Gardner, H., and McCoppin, B. (1988) 'Nursing and politics revisited' in Pittman, E. (ed.) *Shaping Nursing Theory and Practice*. Monograph 1, Lincoln Department of Nursing, La Trobe University 87–107.
Gardner, L. (1968) *The Eye and Ear: The Royal Victorian Eye and Ear Hospital Centenary History* Melbourne: Robertson and Mullens.
Gasson, W. (1980) 'The Evolution of Spectacles: The Chinese Contribution' *The Ophthalmic Optician* Part 1 'Introduction' 5 July: 490–2; Part 2 'The Beginning of Visual Aids' 19 July: 538–46; 'Marco Polo and the Oriental Theory' 2 August: 567–9.
Gibbons, R. (1976a) 'Chiropractic History: Lost, Strayed or Stolen' *American Chiropractors Association Journal of Chiropractic* 13: 18–24.
—— (1976b) Chiropractic in America: The Historical Conflicts of Cultism and Science, unpublished paper presented to 10th DuQuesne University History Forum.
—— (1977) Physician-Chiropractors: Medical Presence in the Evolution of Chiropractic, unpublished paper presented to 50th Annual Meeting of the American Association for History of Medicine, Wisconsin, May.
—— (1980) 'The Rise of the Chiropractic Educational Establishment' in Lints-Dzaman, F. (ed.) *Who's Who in Chiropractic International* Littleton, Colorado: Chiropractic International Publishing Co: 339–51.
Giddens, A. (1971) *Capitalism and Modern Social Theory* London: Cambridge University Press.
—— (1973) *The Class Structure of the Advanced Societies* London: Hutchinson.
Gillison, J. (1974) *Colonial Doctor and His Town* Melbourne: Cypress Books.
Glasner, A.H. (1979) 'Professional Power and State Intervention in Medical Practice' *Australian and New Zealand Journal of Sociology* 15, 3: 20–9.
Goldie, N. (1977) 'The Division of Labour Among Mental Health Professionals: A Negotiated or Imposed Order' in Stacey, M., Reid, M., Heath, C. and Dingwall, R. *Health and the Division of Labour* London: Croom Helm: 141–64.
Goldstein, M. (1975) 'Introduction, Summary and Analysis' in Goldstein, M. (ed.) *The Research Status of Spinal Manipulative Therapy* NINCDS Monograph No. 15: 11–5.
Gorden, R. (1975) *Interviewing Strategy, Techniques and Tactics* Homewood, Ill.: Dorsey.
Gorz, A. (ed.) (1973) *The Division of Labour: The Labour Process and Class Struggle in Modern Capitalism* Sussex: Hassocks.

Gough, I. (1979) *The Political Economy of the Welfare State* London: Macmillan.

Graham, H.B. (1948) 'The Unimaginable Touch of Time: The Centenary of the Royal Melbourne Hospital' *Medical Journal of Australia* 16 August: 213–49.

—— (1952) 'Happenings of the Now Long Past: The Centenary of the Medical Society of Victoria' *Medical Journal of Australia* 16 August: 213–49.

Gramsci, A. (1971) *Prison Notebooks*, edited by Hoare, Q. and Nowell Smith, G. New York: International Publishers.

Gray, W. (1940) 'The History of Optometric Education in Victoria' *Australian Journal of Optometry*: 291–9.

Greenfield, H.I. (with assistance Carol Brown) (1969) *Allied Health Manpower Trends and Prospects* New York: Columbia University Press.

Greenwood, E. (1957) 'Attributes of a Profession' *Social Work* 2, 3: 44–55.

Habermas, J. (1970) 'Technology and Science as "Ideology"' in *Toward a Rational Society* Boston: Beacon Press: 81–122.

—— (1976) *Legitimation Crisis* London: Heinemann.

Hagger, J. (1979) *Colonial Medicine* Adelaide: Rigby.

Hall, S. (1977) 'The Hinterland of Science: Ideology and the "Sociology of Knowledge"' in *On Ideology* Centre for Contemporary Cultural Studies London: Hutchinson: 9–32.

Haug, M.R. (1973) '"Deprofessionalization: An Alternate Hypothesis for the Future' in Halmos, P. (ed.) *Professionalization and Social Change* Sociological Review Monograph No. 20, Keele: 195–210.

—— (1975) 'The Deprofessionalisation of Everyone?' *Sociological Focus* 8 August: 197–213.

Hicks, N. (1978) *This Sin and Scandal* Canberra: Australian National University Press.

—— (1982) 'Medical History and History of Medicine' in Osborne, G. and Mandle, W. *New History: Studying Australia Today* Sydney: Allen & Unwin.

Holloway, S.W.F. (1966) 'The Apothecaries Act 1815: A Reinterpretation' *Medical History* 10, 3: 221–36.

Horobin, G. and McIntosh, J. (1977) 'Responsibility in General Practice' in Stacey, M., Reid, M., Heath, C. and Dingwall, R. *Health and the Division of Labour* London: Croom Helm: 88–114.

Hughes, D. (1977) 'Everyday and Medical Knowledge in Categorizing Patients' in Dingwall, R., Health, C., Reid, M. and Stacey, M. (eds) *Health Care and Health Knowledge* London: Croom Helm: 127–40.

Hughes, E. (1958) *Men and Their Work* Glencoe, Ill.: Free Press.

Illich, I. (1976) *Limits to Medicine* London: Marion Boyars.

Inglis, B. (1964) *Fringe Medicine* London: Faber & Faber.

—— (1978) *The Book of the Back* London: Embury Press.

Inglis, K. (1958) *Hospital and Community: A History of the Royal Melbourne Melbourne Hospital* Melbourne: Melbourne University Press.

International College of Chiropractic/Australian Chiropractors' Association/ Preston Institute of Technology (1979) A Submission to the Victorian Minister for Health, the Honourable W.A. Borthwick MP, Requesting the

Government's Assistance in Obtaining a Grant for Chiropractic Education for 1980–81, ACA Archives.

Jabara, E. (1941a) 'Concept of Optometry' *Australian Journal of Optometry* 31 October: 435–53.

—— (1941b) 'Address to the First General Meeting of the Australian College of Optometry' *Australian Journal of Optometry* 30 May: 219–36.

—— (1942) '1941–1942 Review of the Australian College of Optometry' *Australian Journal of Optometry* 30 June: 260–77.

Jacobs, H. (1926) 'The Causes and Prevention of Maternal Morbidity and Mortality' Part I: *Medical Journal of Australia* 29 May: 593–611; *Medical Journal of Australia* 5 June: 627–43.

James, J.S. (1969) *The Vagabond Papers* Melbourne: Melbourne University Press.

Jamieson, J. (1885) 'A Sketch of the History of Midwifery' *Australian Medical Journal* 15 May: 193–206.

Jamous, J. and Peloille, B. (1970) 'Professions or Self Perpetuating Systems? Changes in the French University Hospital System' in Jackson, J. (ed.) *Professions and Professionalisation* Cambridge: Cambridge University Press: 102–52.

Jewson, N.D. (1976) 'The Disappearance of the Sick-Man from Medical Cosmology' *Sociology* 10: 225.

Johnson, T. (1972) *Professions and Power* London: Macmillan.

—— (1977a) 'The Professions in the Class Structure' in Scase, R. (ed.) *Industrial Society: Class Cleavage and Control* London: Allen & Unwin: 93–110.

—— (1977b) 'What is to be Known: The Structural Determination of Social Class' *Economy and Society* 6, 2: 194–223.

Kane, R., Olsen, D., Leymaster, C., Woolley, F. and Fisher, F. (1979) 'Manipulating the Patient' *Lancet* 7869, 29 June: 1333–1336.

Kaufman, M. (1971) *Homeopathy in America: The Rise and Fall of a Medical Heresy* Baltimore: John Hopkins Press.

Kelly, W. (1859) *Life in Victoria or Victoria in 1853 and Victoria in 1858* London: Chapman and Hall.

Kennedy, R.T. (1946) 'The Remarkable "Dr" Spencer' *Medical Journal of Australia* 1: 149–52.

Kenny, A.L. (1920) 'The Registration of Sight Testing Opticians' *Medical Journal of Australia* 18 September: 260–1.

Kett, W. (1953) 'The History of Optometry in Australia' *Australian Journal of Optometry* 31 January: 15–30.

Keveston, H.L. (1929) 'Prophylactic Obstetrical Practice: An Account of Seven Hundred and Sixty Eight Confinements with Forceps Delivery in General Practice' *Medical Journal of Australia* 5 January: 14–9.

Kingston, B. (ed.) (1977) *The World Moves Slowly: A Documentary History of Australian Women* Australia: Cassell.

Klegon, D. (1978) 'The Sociology of Professions: An Emerging Perspective' *Sociology of Work and Occupations* 5, 3: 259–83.

Kobrin, F. (1966) 'The American Midwife Controversy: A Crisis of Professionalisation' *Bulletin of the History of Medicine* XL, July–August: 350–63.

Krause, E. (1977) *Power and Illness: The Political Sociology of Health and Medical Care* New York: Elsevier.

Kuhn, A. and Wolpe, A. (1978) *Feminism and Materialism: Women and Modes of Production* London: Routledge & Kegan Paul.

Kuhn, T.S. (1970) *The Structure of Scientific Revolutions* 2nd edn, International Encyclopedia of Unified Science.

——— (1970) 'Reflections on My Critics' in Lakatos, I. and Musgrave, A. (eds) *Criticism and the Growth of Knowledge* Cambridge: Cambridge University Press.

Lakatos, I. (1970) 'Falsification and the Methodology of Scientific Research Programmes' in Lakatos, I. and Musgrave, A. (eds) *Criticism and the Growth of Knowledge* Cambridge: Cambridge University Press: 91–177.

Larkin, G. (1978) 'Medical Dominance and Control: Radiographers in the Division of Labour' *Sociological Review* 26, 4: 843–58.

——— (1981) 'Professional Autonomy and the Opthalmic Optician' *Sociology of Health and Illness* 3, 1: 15–30.

Larson, M. Sarfatti (1977) *The Rise of Professionalism: A Sociological Analysis* Berkeley: University of California Press.

——— (1979) 'Professionalism: Rise and Fall' *International Journal of Health Services* 9, 4: 607–27.

——— (1980) 'Proletarianisation and Educated Labour' *Theory and Society* 9, 1: 131–76.

Laslett, P. (1971) *The World We Have Lost* New York: Charles Scribner's Sons.

Lawson, H. (1970) *Joe Wilson's Mate* Hawthorn: Lloyd O'Neill.

Lee, A.E. (1944) 'The History of Appendicitis in Australia: A Window on Abdominal Surgery' *Medical Journal of Australia* 23 December: 653–9.

Lewis, R. (1978) 'Three Close Men: The Story of O.P.S.M.' *Insight* 32, July. 32, July.

Lloyd, W.E. (1968) *A Hundred Years of Medicine* London: Gerald Duckworth and Co. Ltd.

Lomax, E. (1975) 'Manipulative Therapy: A Historical Perspective from Ancient Times to the Modern Era' in Goldstein, M. (ed.) *The Research Status of Spinal Manipulative Therapy* NINCDS Monograph No. 15.

Lowe, R. (1980a) 'The Ophthalmological Society of Melbourne (1889–1913)' *Australian Journal of Opthalmology* 8, 3: 257–70.

——— (1980b) 'Early Melbourne Eye and Ear Hospitals, and Dr. Turnbull's House at 101 (157) Spring Street' *Australian and New Zealand Journal of Surgery* 50, 5: 546–9.

Lowenstein, W. (ed.) (1978) *Weevils in the Flour: An Oral Record of the 1930's Depression in Australia* Melbourne: Hyland House.

Lupton, G., Najman, J.H. Payne, S., Sheehan, M. and Western, J.S. (1978) 'The Demographic Characteristics of Patients Presenting for Chiropractic and Related Forms of Treatment' *Community Health Studies* 1, 2: 51–6.

McCarthy, P.G. (1970) 'Wages in Australia 1891–1914' *Australian Economic History Review* 10, 1: 56–76.

——— (1972) 'Wages for Unskilled Work and Margins for Skill, Australia 1901–1921' *Australian Economic History Review* 12, 2: 142–60.

McCorkle, T. (1961) 'Chiropractic: A Deviant Theory of Disease and Treat-

ment in Contemporary Western Culture' *Human Organization* 20: 20–2.
Mackay, E.A. (1934) 'Medical Men as Pastoral Pioneers' *Medical Journal of Australia* 2: 476–83.
—— (1936) 'Medical Practice During the Goldfields Era in Victoria' *Medical Journal of Australia* 26 September: 421–8.
McDonough, R. and Harrison, R. (1978) 'Patriarchy and Relations of Production' in Kuhn, A. and Wolpe, A. (eds) *Feminism and Materialism* London: Routledge & Kegan Paul: 11–41.
McKeown, T. (1970) 'A Sociological Approach to the History of Medicine' *Medical History* 14: 342–51.
McKinlay, J. (nd) The Proletarianization of Physicians, unpublished paper, Boston University.
—— (1977) 'The Business of Good Doctoring or Doctoring as Good Business: Reflections on Freidson's View of the Medical Game' *International Journal of Health Services* 7, 3: 458–83.
McKinlay, J. and McKinlay, S. (1977) 'The Questionable Effect of Medical Measures on the Decline of Mortality in the Twentieth Century' *Millbank Memorial Fund Quarterly* 55, 3: 405–28.
Maddox, K. (1937) 'The Influence of Robert Koch on the History of Tuberculosis' *Medical Journal of Australia* 30 October: 801–2.
Mandel, E. (1975) *Late Capitalism* London: New Left Books.
Marcuse, H. (1969) *Negations: Essays in Critical Theory* London: Penguin.
—— (1971) 'Industrialisation and Capitalims' in Stammer, O. (ed.) *Max Weber and Sociology Today* Oxford: Blackwells: 133–86.
Marglin, S. (1974) 'What Do Bosses Do: The Origins and Functions of Hierarchy in Capitalist Production' *Review of Radical Political Economics* 6, 2: 60–112.
Marx, K. (1969) *Capital Vol. IV: Theories of Surplus Value* London: Burns.
—— (1973) *The Poverty of Philosophy* Moscow: Progress Publishers.
—— (1968) *The German Ideology* Moscow: Progress Publishers.
Mechanic, D. (1976) *The Growth of Bureaucratic Medicine* New York: Wiley. York: Wiley.
Mengert, W. (1942) 'The Origins of the Male Midwife' *Annals of Medical History* 4, 5: 453–65.
Merrington, J. (1968) 'Theory and Practice in Gramsci's Marxism' in Miliband, R. and Saville, J. (eds) *Socialist Register* New York: Monthly Review Press: 145–76.
Mickle, D. (1979) *Koo-Wee-Rup: A Brief History of 130 Years* Melbourne: Sun Press.
Miliband, R. (1970) *The State in Capitalist Society* London: Weidenfield and Nicholson.
—— (1973) 'Poulantzas and the Capitalist State' *New Left Review* 82.
Mills, C. Wright (1959) *The Sociological Imagination* New York: Oxford University Press.
Mitchell, A. (1977) *The Hospital South of the Yarra* Melbourne: Alfred Hospital.
Mishra, R. (1979) 'Technology and Social Structure in Marx's Theory: An Exploratory Analysis' *Science and Society* 43, 2: 132–57.
Moore, W. (1970) *The Professions, Rules and Roles* New York: Russell Sage Foundation.

Moran, H.W. (1939) *Viewless Winds, Being the Recollections and Digressions of an Australian Surgeon* London: Peter Davies.

Morris, E.S: (1925) 'An Essay on the Causes and Prevention of Maternal Morbidity and Mortality' *Medical Journal of Australia* 12 September 301-44.

Musgrove, F. (1959) 'Middle-Class Education and Employment in the Nineteenth Century' *Economic History Review* 12 August: 99-111.

Nathan, J. (1980) 'Kurrajong People and Crystal Balls' *Australian Journal of Optometry* 63, 4: 164-8.

Navarro, V. (1976) *Medicine Under Capitalism* New York: Prodist.

—— (1980) 'Work, Ideology and Science' *Social Science and Medicine* 14c: 191-205.

Newman, C. (1957) *The Evolution of Medical Education in the Nineteenth Century* Oxford: Oxford University Press.

Nisbet, W.B. (1891) 'The Education of Midwives' *Australasian Medical Gazette* June: 269-71.

Oakley, A. (1976) "Wisewoman and Medicine Man: Changes in the Management of Childbirth' in Mitchell, J. and Oakley, A. (eds) *The Rights and Wrongs of Women* Harmondsworth: Penguin: 17-58.

O'Boyle, L. (1970) 'The Problems of an Excess of Educated Men in Western Europe 1800-1850' *Journal of Modern History* 4, 42: 471-95.

O'Connor, J. (1973) *The Fiscal Crisis of the State* New York: St. Martins Press.

Offe, C. (1972) "Political Authority and Class Structures: An Analysis of State Capitalist Societies' *International Journal of Sociology* 2, 1: 73-108.

Oppenheimer, M. (1973) 'The Proletarianisation of the Professional' in Halmos, P. (ed.) *Professionalisation and Social Change* Sociological Review Monograph No. 20: 213-28.

O'Malley, P. (1979) 'Theories of Structure Versus Causal Determination: Accounting for Legislative Change in Capitalist Societies' in Tomasic, R. (ed.) *Legislation and Society in Australia* Sydney: Law Foundation of NSW; Allen & Unwin: 50-65.

Parker, G. and Tupling, H. (1976) 'The Chiropractic Patient: Psychological Aspects' *Medical Journal of Australia* 4 September: 373-76.

—— (1977a) 'On Going to a Chiropractor' Appendix 10, *Report of the Committee of Inquiry into Chiropractic, Osteopathy, Homeopathy and Naturopathy* (known as Parker Report No. 1) Canberra: Australian Government Publishing Service: 571-99.

—— (1977b) 'Consumer Evaluation of Natural Therapies' Appendix 11, *Report of the Committee of Inquiry into Chiropractic, Osteopathy, Homeopathy and Naturopathy* (known as Parker Report No. 2) Canberra: Australian Government Publishing Service: 600-22.

Parker, G., Tupling, H. and Pryor, D. (1978) 'A Controlled Trial of Cervical Manipulation for Migraine' *Australian and New Zealand Journal of Medicine* December.

Parkin, F. (1974) *The Social Analysis of Class Structure* London: Tavistock.

—— (1979) *Marxism and Class Theory: A Bourgeois Critique* London: Tavistock.

Parry, N. and Parry, J. (1976) *The Rise of the Medical Profession* London: Croom Helm.

Parsons, T. (1964) *The Social System* New York: Free Press.
—— (1968) 'Professions' in *International Encyclopaedia of Social Sciences* New York: 534–46.
Pellissier, J. (1979) Childbirth in Victoria Before 1900, unpublished paper, Department of Sociology, Monash University.
Pensabene, T. (1980) *The Rise of the Medical Practitioner in Victoria* Research Monograph No. 2, Health Research Project, Canberra: Australian National University.
Peterson, M.J. (1978) *The Medical Profession in Mid-Victorian London* Berkeley: University of California Press.
Popper, K. (1959) *The Logic of Scientific Discovery* London: Hutchinson.
Posner, T. (1977) 'Magical Elements in Orthodox Medicine' in Dingwall, R., Heath, C., Reid, M. and Stacey, M. (eds) *Health Care and Health Knowledge* London: Croom Helm: 141–59.
Potter, J. (1981) 'Cancer—Nineteenth Century Science—Twentieth Century Technology' *Community Health Studies* V, 2: 133–41.
Potter, W.L. (1938) 'Anaesthetics in Australia in the Early Days' *Medical Journal of Australia* 3 December: 940–9.
Poulantzas, N. (1973) *Political Power and Social Classes* London: New Left Books.
—— (1975) *Classes in Contemporary Capitalism* London: New Left Books.
—— (1978) *State, Power and Socialism* London: New Left Books.
Powles, J. (1973) 'On the Limitations of Modern Medicine' *Science, Medicine and Man* 1, 1: 1–30.
Pownall, E. (1964) *Australian Pioneer Women* 3rd edn, Adelaide: Rigby.
Prendergast, J. (1968) *Pioneers of the Omeo District* Melbourne: Riall.
Preston Institute of Technology (1978) A Submission on Chiropractic Course Siting to the Ad Hoc Committee on Chiropractic of the VIC, ACA Archives, December.
Pringle, R. (1973) 'Octavious Beale and the Ideology of the Birth Rate: The Royal Commissions of 1904 and 1905' *Refractory Girl* Winter: 19–27.
Przeworski, A. (1977) 'The Process of Class Formation from Karl Kautsky's *The Class Struggle* to Recent Debates' *Politics and Society* 7, 4: 343–402.
Purdy, J. (1921) 'Maternal Mortality in Childbirth' *Medical Journal of Australia* 15 January: 39–45.
Quinney, R. (1970) *The Social Reality of Crime* New York: Little Brown.
Radcliffe, W. (1967) *Milestones in Midwifery* Bristol: Wright and Sons.
Reader, W.J. (1966) *Professional Men: The Rise of the Professional Classes in Nineteenth Century England* London: Weidenfield & Nicholson.
Reeves, C.E. (1861) 'Fighting Doctors' *Medical Record of Australia* 1 December: 135–6.
Renaud, M. (1975) 'On the Structural Constraints to State Intervention in Health' *International Journal of Health Services* 5, 4: 559–71.
Rich, A. (1976) *Of Woman Born: Motherhood as Experience and Institution* London: Virago.
Richardson, J. (1984) 'An economic perspective on Chiropractic in Australia' in Campbell, S.A., Dillon, J.L., and Jamison, J. *Proceedings of a Conference on Development and Needs in Education and Social Science Research of Chiropractic* Armidale: University of New England 98–128.

—— (1988) 'Complementary healers' forthcoming in Najman, J. and Lupton, G. (ed) *Health and Australian Society: some Sociological Perspectives* Macmillan.

Robertson, A.P.L. (1858) *Medical Reform: An Enquiry into the Relation Existing Between the Public and the Profession* Melbourne: Fairfax.

Rodberg, L. and Stevenson, G. (1977) 'The Health Care Industry in Advanced Capitalism' *Review of Radical Political Economy* 9, 1: 104–15.

Roe, M. (1976/7) 'The Establishment of the Australian Department of Health: Its Background and Significance' *Historical Studies* 17: 176–92.

Rose, H. and Rose, S. (1969) *Science and Society* London: Allen Lane.

Rose, S. (1977) 'Science and Capitalism' *New Left Review* 61: 2–13.

Rosen, G. (1944) *The Specialization of Medicine with Particular Reference to Ophthalmology* New York: Froben.

—— (1973) 'Health, History and the Social Sciences' *Social Science and Medicine* 7, April: 233–48.

Rosenberg, C. (1971) 'The Medical Profession, Medical Practice and the History of Medicine; in Clarke, E. (ed.) *Modern Methods in the History of Medicine* London: Althone: 22–35.

Rosenthal, N. (1974) *People Not Cases: The Royal District Nursing Service* Melbourne: Nelson.

Roth, J. (1957) 'Ritual and Magic in the Control of Contagion' *American Sociological Review* 22, June: 310–4.

Rothstein, W. (1972) *American Physicians in the Nineteenth Century: From Sects to Science* Baltimore: John Hopkins University Press.

Royal Women's Hospital, Melbourne (1962) *Centenary of Nurse Training in Australia, 1862–1962* Melbourne.

Rueschmeyer, D. (1973) 'Doctors and Lawyers: A Comment on the Theory of the Professions' *Canadian Review of Sociology and Anthropology* 1, February: 17–30.

Russell, K. (1977) *The Melbourne Medical School, 1862–1972* Melbourne: Melbourne University Press.

Sands and McDougall (1903–1909) *Directory of Victoria*.

Sax, S. (1972) *Medical Care in the Melting Pot* Sydney: Angus and Robertson.

Sayers, C.E. (1956) *The Women's ... A Social History* Melbourne: Pride.

Schudson, M. (1980) 'Review of Larson's "Rise of Professionalism"' *Theory and Society* 9, 1: 215–29.

Scotton, R. (1974) *Medical Care in Australia: An Economic Diagnosis* Melbourne: Sun Books.

Scull, A. (1975) 'From Madness to Mental Illness: Medical Men as Moral Entrepreneurs' *European Journal of Sociology*, 16, 2, 218–261.

Segall, M. (1977) The Political Economy of Doctors' Social Practice, unpublished paper quoted in Robson, J. 'Quality, Inequality and Health Care' *Medicine in Society* April: 19.

Shaw, W.F. (1947) 'Development of Obstetrics and Gynaecology' *Medical Journal of Australia* 6 September: 285–9.

Shyrock. R.H. (1948) *The Development of Modern Medicine: An Interpretation of the Social and Scientific Factors Involved* London: Gollancz.

Interpretation of the Social and Scientific Factors Involved London:

Sigerist, H. (1951) *A History of Medicine* New York: Oxford University Press.

—— (1960) 'The History of Medical Licensure' in Roemer, M.I. (ed.) *Henry E. Sigerist on the Sociology of Medicine* New York: M.D. Publications: 308–18.

Sinclair, W.A. (1975) 'Economic Growth and Well Being, Melbourne, 1870–1914' *Economic Record* 51: 153–73.

Siskind, M., Lupton, G., Sheehan, M., Burns, V., Najman, J.M. and Western, J.S. (1977) 'The Patient's View of Chiropractic: A Brisbane Study' in *Report of Committee of Inquiry into Chiropractic, Osteopathy, Homeopathy and Naturopathy* (Western Report No. 4) Canberra: Australian Government Publishing Service: 523–70.

Skipper, J. (1978) 'Medical Sociology and Chiropractic' *Sociological Symposium* 22: 1–5.

Skirving, R.S. (1932) 'Fifty Years in a Changing World: The British Medical Association in Australia' *Medical Journal of Australia* 23 July: 99–104.

Smith, J. (ed.) (1903) *The Cyclopedia of Victoria* Volume I, Melbourne: Cyclopedia.

Smith, R.L. (1969) *At Your Own Risk: The Case Against Chiropractic* New York: Trident Press.

Stawell, R.K. (1931) 'The Halford Oration: The Foundation of a Medical School and the Progress of Medical Education' *Medical Journal of Australia* 3 January: 1–8.

Stevens, R. (1966) *Medical Practice in Modern England* New Haven: Yale University Press.

Stone, L. (1977) *The Family, Sex and Marriage in England, 1500–1800* London: Weidenfied & Nicholson.

Sumner, C. (1979) *Reading Ideologies: An Investigation into the Marxist Theory of Ideology and Law* London: Academic Press.

Summers, A. (1975) *Damned Whores and God's Police* Ringwood: Penguin.

Sutcliffe, G. (1950) 'Brief Survey of the Optometrical Profession in Victoria' *Australian Journal of Optometry* 30 November: 490–3.

Swingewood, A. (1975) *Marx and Modern Society Theory* London: Macmillan.

Szasz, T. (1971) *The Manufacture of Madness* London: Routledge & Kegan Paul.

Teale, R. (ed.) (1978) *Colonial Eve: Sources of Women in Australia, 1788–1914* Melbourne: Oxford University Press.

Templeton, J. (1969) *Prince Henry's: The Evolution of a Melbourne Hospital 1869–1969* Melbourne: Robertson & Mullens.

Thatcher, C. (1864) *Colonial Minstrel* Melbourne.

Therborn, G. (1976) *Science, Class and Society: On the Formation of Sociology and Historical Materialism* London: New Left Books.

Thornton, A. (1972) 'The Past in Midwifery Services' *Australian Nurses Journal* 1: 19–23.

Townsend, L. (1952) 'Obstetrics Through the Ages' *Medical Journal of Australia* 26 April: 557–65.

Trinca, A. (1931) Quackery and Its Effects on the Health of the Community: Lecture to members Royal Victorian Trained Nurses Association, 18 August, AMA Archives.

Victorian Women's Health Policy Working Group (1987) *Why Women's*

Health?: Victorian Women Respond Melbourne: Victorian Government Publishing Service.

Versluysen, M.C. (1981) 'Midwives, Medical Men and "Poor Women Labouring of Child"': Lying' in Hospitals in Eighteenth Century London' in Roberts, J. (ed.) *Women, Health and Reproduction* London: Routledge & Kegan Paul: 18–49.

Waddington, I. (1977) 'General Practitioners and Consultants in Early Nineteenth Century England: The Sociology of Intra-Professional Conflict' in Woodward, J. and Richards, D. (eds) *Health Care and Popular Medicine in Nineteenth Century England* London: Croom Helm: 164–88.

Ward, R. (1978) *The Australian Legend* Melbourne: Oxford University Press.

Wardwell, W.I. (1952) 'A Marginal Professional Role: The Chiropractor' *Social Forces* 30: 339–48.

—— (1972) 'Orthodoxy and Heterodoxy in Medical Practice' *Social Science and Medicine* 6: 759–63.

—— (1976) 'Orthodox and Unorthodox Practitioners: Changing Relationships and Future Status of Chiropractors' in Wallis, R. and Morley, P. (eds) *Marginal Medicine* New York: Free Press: 61–73.

—— (1978) 'Social Factors in the Survival of Chiropractic: A Comparative View' *Sociological Symposium* 22: 6–17.

Waterman, B. and Waitzkin, H. (1977) 'Ideology and Social Control in the Doctor Patient Relationship' *Ideology in Medicine* HMO Packet No. 4: 42–70.

Weber, M. (1947) *The Theory of Social and Economic Organisation* Glencoe: Free Press.

—— (1968) *Economy and Society* Volume III New York: Bedminster Press.

Webster, M.E. (1942) 'The History of the Trained Nurse in Victoria' *Victorian Historical Magazine* 19, 4: 121–32.

Weisz, G. (1978) 'The Politics of Medical Professionalisation' *Journal of Social History* 12, 1: 3–30.

Wheelwright, E. (1976) 'Introduction' in Wheelwright, E. and Buckley, K. *Essays in the Political Economy of Australian Capitalism* Volume 1 Sydney: Australia and New Zealand Book Company: 1–11.

White, M. and Skipper, J. (1972) 'The Chiropractic Physician: A Study of the Career Contingencies of a Marginal Occupation' *The Journal of Clinical Chiropractic* Archive Edition II, Winter: 148–55.

Williams, D. (1947) 'Eyes, Surgeons and Sociality in Australasia' *Trans. Ophthalmol. Soc. Aust.* 7, 5.

—— (1953) 'A Review of Some of the Affairs of the Ophthalmological Society of Victoria (BMA)' *Trans. Ophtalmol. Soc. Aust.* 13: 19–34.

Willcox, S., and Ednie, G. (1987) 'Critique of the Health Service (Conciliation and Review) Bill' *Health Issues* No 9, March.

Willis, E. (1978a) 'Alternative Medicine and the Struggle for Legitimacy: Consequences for the Consumer' *New Doctor* 9, August: 15–18.

—— (1978b) 'Professionalism and Bureaucracy: The Changing Context of Primary Medical Care' *Community Health Studies* 2, 1 October: 1–12.

—— (1979) 'Sister Elizabeth Kenny and the Evolution of the Occupational Division of Labour in Health Care' *Australian and New Zealand Journal of Sociology*, 15, 3: 30–38.

—— (1982) 'Research and Teaching in the Sociology of Health and Illness in Australia and New Zealand' *Community Health Studies* 6, 2: 144–53.

Willis, E. and Willis (Wyn) J. (1981) Hands of Flesh, Hands of Iron: Class and Gender in the Historical Transformation of Attendance at Childbirth, unpublished paper, SAANZ Conference, Christchurch, New Zealand.

Winer, C. (1977) 'Manipulative Medicine Versus Chiropractic' *Australian Medical Association Gazette* 8 December.

Winter, D. (1975) A Submission on Chiropractic by the Australian Chiropractic Association to the Federal Committee of Inquiry into Chiropractic, Osteopathy and Naturopathy.

Woodward, J. and Richards, D. (1977) 'Toward a Social History of Medicine' in Woodward, J. and Richards, D. (eds) *Health Care and Popular Medicine in Nineteenth Century England* London: Croom Helm: 15–55.

Worrall, R. (1909) 'The Necessity for Organisation in the Profession' *Intercolonial Medical Journal of Australia* 20 December: 585–98.

Wright, C. (1979) 'Sixty Years of Optometry' *Australian Journal of Optometry* 62: published in five parts. No. 1, January: 20–3; No. 3, March: 108–13; No. 4, April: 158–60; No. 5, May: 203–9; No. 6, June: 252–55.

—— (1980a) 'The History of Optometric Research in Australia' *Australian Journal of Optometry* 63, 4: 149–63.

—— (1980b) 'Opening Address for the Golden Jubilee Congress of the Australian Optometrical Association' *Australian Journal of Optometry* November: 4.

Wright, E.O. (1978) *Class, Crisis and the State* London: New Left Books.

—— (1980a) 'Alternative Perspectives on the Marxist Concept of Class' *Politics and Society* 9, 3: 323–70.

—— (1980b) 'Class and Occupation' *Theory and Society* 9, 1: 177–214.

Zwar, B.T. (1946) 'The Royal Melbourne Hospital: Some Milestones in its Development' *Royal Melbourne Hospital Clinical Reports* 17, December: 7–10.

Index

Andrew, R., 174, 181
Armstrong, D., 22, 209
Armstrong, M., 67
Atkinson, P., 4
Australian Chiropractors Association, 171, 173, 180–190, 194
Australian Medical Association, 3, 19, 32, 176, 180–7, 190, 207, 215
Australian Physiotherapy Association, 183–4

Barrett, M., 18, 123
Berlant, G., 11
Berliner, H., 22–3, 82–3, 86, 90, 208
Bowden, K., 42, 48–50, 102
Bucher, R., 4–5, 45
Brown, E.R., 23–5, 82, 208
Browne, D., 117

Cambridge, A., 100
Campbell, J., 121–2
capitalism, 5; changes in, 111
chemists, 44–5
class, 14; health occupations and, 13, 17, 202; struggle, 6, 17; and the state, 26–7; and gender, 123
Cochrane, A., 209

Davies, C., 4, 30
Davison, G., 47, 60
Deising, P., 213
Dillon, R., 199
Donnison, J., 95–7, 122
Duke-Elder, S., 133
Durkheim, E., 9, 205

Figlio, K., 21, 211–12

Forbes, T., 95
Forster, F., 99, 101–4, 106
Frankenberg, R., 10
Freidson, E., 4, 9–10, 16, 19–20, 23, 31, 54, 64–5, 204, 206–7, 209, 211
Friendly Societies, 75–7

Gamarnikow, E., 18, 204
Gandevia, B., 41, 44–6, 49, 55, 67
gender, 17–8, 123, 205
Gibbons, R., 167–9
Gillison, J., 101
Goldie, N., 31
Gorden, R., 213
Gramsci, A., 16

Habermas, G., 16, 20–1, 28, 34
Hart, A., 176–7
Haug, M., 209
Hicks, N., 109, 211
homeopathy, 23, 58–60, 73
Hughes, E., 32

ideology, 8; professionalism as, 8; scientific medicine and, 19–20; 25, 198
Illich, I., 26, 33
Inglis, B., 165, 198
Inglis, K., 45, 63

Jabara, E., 152–3
Jacobs, H., 120
James, J., 71
Jamous, J., 23, 208
Johnson, T., 9, 10–1, 14–6, 75, 91, 206

Kelly, W., 43-4
Kett, W., 138-9, 146, 155
Klegon, D., 46
Kobrin, F., 99
Krause, E., 33
Kuhn, T., 21, 61-3, 81

Larkin, G., 4, 32, 128, 161, 203, 207
Larson, M.S., 11-2, 25, 38, 42,
    46-7, 62, 78
Lawson, H., 71
Lewis, R., 147-8
Lomax, E., 165-6
Lowe, R., 134-5
Lowenstein, W., 118

McCorkle, T., 170
McGrath, A., 45, 56
Mackay, E., 37-40
McKinlay, J., 4-5, 10, 207
Mandel, E., 34
Marglin, S., 34
Marx, K., 9, 205
Melbourne Medical School, 54,
    82-9, 104-5, 151-2
Mishra, R., 24
Musgrove, F., 39

Navarro, V., 12-3, 25, 29, 35, 91
N.Z. report on chiropractic, 192-3

Oakley, A., 98
O'Connor, J., 28
OPSM, 127-9, 147-9, 159

Palmer, B., 168-9
Palmer, D., 166-7
Parker, G., 188, 193-4, 200
Parsons, T., 9, 17
Parry, N. & Parry, J., 11, 30
Pellissier, J., 117
Peloille, B., 23, 208
Pensabene, T., 121, 45-6, 55-7, 60,
    62-4, 69, 73, 76-7, 80, 104
Peterson, M.J., 25, 37-40, 78, 133
Popper, K., 21
Poulantzas, N., 14, 26-7
Powles, J., 66
Pownall, E., 100

Prendergast, J., 101
professionalism, 8-13, 16, 25, 119
Przeworki, A., 14, 18

Rich, A., 94
Roberts, F., 172
Rockefeller Foundation, 82, 87-9
Rose, S. & Rose, H., 19
Rosen, G., 32, 132
Rosenberg, C., 62
Rosenthal, N., 106, 118
Roth, J., 19, 111
Rothstein, W., 22, 65
Royal Melbourne Institute of
    Technology, 182, 188-9
Russell, K., 54-5, 62, 83-5

Sairey Gamp, 100-1, 107
Sax, S., 33
Scull, A., 35
Segall, M., 26
Smith, D., 156
State, 5-6, 26-30, 202-3
Strauss, A., 4-5, 45

Teale, R., 100
technological determinism, 5, 33-5,
    61, 201-2, 204-5
Templeton, J., 58-9, 80
Thame, C., 113, 119
Thatcher, C., 44
Tupling, A., 188, 193-4, 200

United Chiropractors Association,
    171, 179, 185

Versluysen, M., 17-8, 94-5, 97-8

Waitzkin, H., 20
Wardwell, W., 167, 169
Waterman, B., 20
Weber, M., 9, 205
Wells, C., 172-3, 176
Wheelwright, E., 28-9
Williams, D., 133, 135, 141, 147,
    155
Wright, C., 136
Wright, E.O., 13-4, 17, 212, 214

Printed in the United States
by Baker & Taylor Publisher Services

Printed in the United States
by Baker & Taylor Publisher Services